MAP:
The Co-Creative
White Brotherhood
Medical Assistance Program

SECOND EDITION

MAP

THE CO-CREATIVE
WHITE BROTHERHOOD
MEDICAL
ASSISTANCE
PROGRAM

MACHAELLE SMALL WRIGHT

PERELANDRA, LTD.

CENTER FOR NATURE RESEARCH

JEFFERSONTON ℐ VIRGINIA

This book is manufactured in the United States of America.
Designed by Machaelle Small Wright.
Cover design by James F. Brisson, Williamsville, VT 05362.
Editing by David and Machaelle Small Wright.
Copyediting by Elizabeth McHale, Williamsburg, MA 01096.
Production assistance by Clarence N. Wright.
Formatting, typesetting, and computer wizardry
by Machaelle Small Wright.

This book was formatted, laid out, and produced
using the Xerox Ventura Publisher software along with
the Hewlett Packard Laser Jet 4 printer.

Printed on recycled paper.

Published by Perelandra, Ltd.,
P.O. Box 3603, Warrenton, VA 20188

Library of Congress Card Catalog Number: 94-065465
Wright, Machaelle Small
MAP: The Co-Creative White Brotherhood
Medical Assistance Program

ISBN 0-927978-19-9

89

Contents

Preface

The Light at
the End of the Tunnel
by Albert Schatz, Ph.D.*

This is an extraordinary book. To do it justice, I
would like to begin by putting it in proper
perspective. Man's localized destruction of nature has
been responsible for the extinction of many animal
species. Now our global assault on nature threatens *our*
survival. Instead of implementing Franklin Delano
Roosevelt's Four Freedoms, we have chosen a collision
course with the Four Horsemen of the Apocalypse. Individuals who exhibit such self-destructive behavior are
considered to be mentally deranged. But, like Thespians
in a Greek tragedy, "merrily we go to hell."

We are running out of natural resources, out of natural
environment, out of space, and out of time. In our
suicidal assault on nature, we are approaching the point
of no return. The world's military budget is a barometer,

* *Dr. Schatz discovered the antibiotic Streptomycin, which was the first effective
means of treating human tuberculosis. For this and other research, he received
honorary degrees and medals, and was named an honorary member of scientific,
medical, and dental societies in Europe, Latin America, and the U.S.*

odometer, and speedometer of our mad rush to oblivion. The arms race turns out to have been a race to annihilation. The insanity of Vietnam has metastasized into global insanity. In Vietnam, "we had to destroy a city in order to save it." Now we are destroying the world— allegedly to save it in one way or another, for one purpose or another. The wages of this sin were pointed out by Dwight Eisenhower in his 1953 Cross of Iron speech.

> . . . *Every gun that is made, every warship launched, every rocket fired signifies, in the final sense, a theft from those who hunger and are not fed, those who are cold and are not clothed.*
>
> *This world in arms is not spending money alone.*
>
> *It is spending the sweat of its laborers, the genius of its scientists, the hopes of its children.*
>
> *The cost of one modern heavy bomber is this: a modern brick school in more than thirty cities. . . .*
>
> *We pay for a single fighter plane with a half million bushels of wheat.*
>
> *We pay for a single destroyer with new homes that could have housed more than eight thousand people.*
>
> *This, I repeat, is the best way of life to be found on the road the world has been taking.*
>
> *This is not a way of life at all, in any true sense. Under the cloud of threatening war, it is humanity hanging from a cross of iron. . . .*

We obviously will not be saved by our anthropocentric science, which has given us chemical dumps, deadly radioactive waste that we do not know how to dispose of, air and water pollution, carcinogenic pesticides and food additives, ineffective and harmful synthetic drugs, nerve gas, nuclear weapons, biological warfare, the profligate waste of natural resources, the global devastation of nature, and much more. This is what science means to many people. We obviously also will not be saved by academic scientists whose research is supported by grants from and, in turn, supports the pharmaceutical, agricultural, and chemical industries—and the military. Indeed, the military-industrial complex that Eisenhower warned us about has metastasized into a military-industrial-educational complex.

YE SHALL KNOW THE TRUTH
AND THE TRUTH SHALL MAKE YOU FREE

Where can we go from here? Is there a way out? I am convinced that our only salvation is what Machaelle Small Wright calls "co-creative science." This involves our consciously establishing a co-creative partnership with nature. But before we do that, we should know what nature is and who we are with respect to nature.

This and other essential information is now readily available as a result of research that Machaelle has done in collaboration with nature. Her published reports are not merely descriptive narratives of devas, nature spirits, and other intelligences. Instead, they provide us with clear definitions and a simple hands-on approach so we know how and with whom we can communicate and work. Moreover, we can all engage in co-creative science and work in a co-creative partnership with nature, *if* we want to. It is not necessary that we take courses in biology, chemistry, physics, geology, calculus, etc., and get degrees. The only credentials we need are intent, sincerity, commitment, and the information and processes available in Perelandra publications.

Co-creative science is qualitatively different from the science we know because it integrates the involutionary input of nature (order, organization, and life vitality/action) with the evolutionary dynamic of man (direction and purpose). Until now, science has been essentially evolutionary. (These and other terms are defined in Machaelle's publications.) Co-creative science is therefore not a linear advance over present-day science, but it is qualitatively unique. It was developed *de novo* in the sense that it is not derived from contemporary science. It employs different methodologies and obtains information from sources with which contemporary science has never worked. Co-creative science may be graphically represented, using the "V" diagram shown on the next page.

I believe that co-creative science is the science of the future, that it will revolutionize our understanding of science, philosophy, and psychology; and that it will provide us with a new kind of agriculture and new ways of achieving health.

This leads directly to Machaelle's book—*MAP: The Co-Creative White Brotherhood Medical Assistance Program*. All of us are concerned with health. But what is health? And

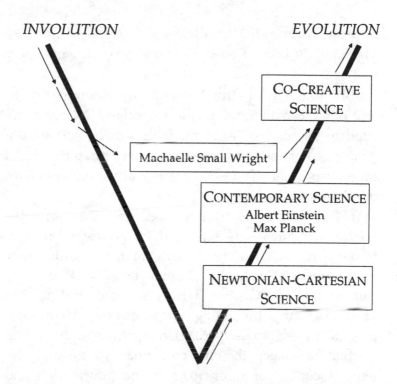

INVOLUTION

EVOLUTION

CO-CREATIVE
SCIENCE

Machaelle Small Wright

CONTEMPORARY SCIENCE
Albert Einstein
Max Planck

NEWTONIAN-CARTESIAN
SCIENCE

Newtonian-Cartesian Science, also known as Classical Science, developed in the 17th century. That science was based on the work of the physicist Sir Isaac Newton and the philosopher René Descartes. Contemporary, present-day science is based on the research of Max Planck, "the father of quantum mechanics" (1900), and Albert Einstein's theories of relativity (1905 and 1916).

how is it best achieved, supported, and maintained? Unfortunately, there is something wrong with how these questions are answered. While we have been bombarded with more and more information on health, our health has been declining. While we have been spending more and more money on health, we have become more and more unhealthy. Obviously, what we need is a new approach, one that will be effective. *MAP*, like Machaelle's book *Flower Essences*, provides precisely that.

MAP is not allopathy, homeopathy, naturopathy, or any other conventional medical specialty. Nor is it related to alternative health modalities or holistic health. And it is not esoteric, occult, new age, or spiritual. All those approaches to health are essentially evolutionary developments by man.

MAP is qualitatively different because, like co-creative science of which it is a part, it integrates the involutionary input of nature with man's evolutionary development. The healthy human being is a balanced combination of these two dynamics. We do not need to know anatomy, physiology, biochemistry, pathology, psychology, etc., to use MAP effectively. As in the case of co-creative science, the only credentials we need are intent, sincerity, commitment, and the information and processes in Machaelle's book.

But *MAP* offers much more than health *per se*. Like Machaelle's other books, *MAP* also increases our understanding of who and what we are, what nature and reality are, what our place in the universe is, what our responsibilities are, and what amazing opportunities we have.

Machaelle's co-creative research with nature is not only the light at the end of the tunnel. It is also the entrance to the tunnel and the tunnel itself.

M A P :
The Co-Creative
White Brotherhood
Medical Assistance Program

L'Chaim

Chapter 1

Some Personal Comments and How MAP Was Developed

In 1982, my work expanded in ways that were both exhilarating and extremely challenging. Since 1976, I had been working exclusively with nature intelligences in research dedicated to developing a working partnership between humans and nature. But in 1982, I learned from nature that I could expand the research in a way that would link it directly into the activities of an organization called the "White Brotherhood." I also learned that this connection was beneficial to nature and to us, as well as to the White Brotherhood. So, I decided to do it.

This decision set off a chain of events that, among other things, led me into a whole new level of understanding of the human body and its relationship to the soul. You see, my decision to expand the research at Perelandra was a soul decision. Once the decision was made, I discovered that implementing it depended on my ability to physically hold, support, and process all

1

that the expansion required of me. I had understood something about this relationship between the soul and the body for years, but the 1982 expansion brought it into a new and more intense light.

Usually, when I've discussed this situation with others, they immediately think that the thing one must do in order to meet the challenges of expansion is change the diet. Over the years, I've realized how much we lean on diet as a solution for everything. Well, I never changed my diet nor, after much questioning, was I ever instructed to change my diet. The eating patterns that I had established prior to 1982 were sufficient for what I was faced with after 1982. If diet wasn't the answer to my functioning well on this more expanded level of the nature research, then I would have to find other answers.

To help you to understand the scope of the expansion I am talking about and why it presented challenges, let me give you a thumbnail description of the White Brotherhood and nature intelligences. After all, if you decide to enter the MAP program, you will be working with them as well and I'm sure you'd appreciate knowing who they are. Before you get nervous, however, and think that your working with them will necessitate your dealing with the kinds of challenges I encountered, let me assure you that this will not be the case. I had to expand myself into the dimension of the White Brotherhood in order to work with them on a daily basis in a working team relationship. This has impacted the scope, quality, direction, and expression of the Perelandra work. Your expansion will center around your decision to work with the White Brotherhood and nature in areas involving your health and personal balance. You will not have to expand into another dimension. In short, the White Brotherhood and nature team will be making "house calls."

THE WHITE BROTHERHOOD

I became aware of the White Brotherhood's link with the research at Perelandra in 1980. For two years, I ignored them while I maintained my focus exclusively on nature intelligences and our work. I figured that whatever connection the White Brotherhood had would be best handled by them and they didn't need me. Besides, at that time, I knew next to nothing about them and had no desire to know more.

Much has been written about the White Brotherhood, but I think a lot of it was garbage. Some people have felt or said that they were the sole "channellers" of the White Brotherhood, and this simply isn't true. The Brotherhood is a huge organization that is constantly connected to us in general and to many of us individually. It's just that usually they are only able to work with us on an intuitive level, and our link with them is unconscious on our part.

The White Brotherhood is a large group of highly evolved souls dedicated to assisting the evolutionary process of moving universal reality, principles, laws, and patterns through all planes and levels of form. They hold the major patterning and rhythms now being utilized for the shift we are all going through from the Piscean to the Aquarian era. When we link with them, they support and assist us by assuring that any work we do maintains its forward evolutionary motion and its connection to the new Aquarian dynamics.

They exist beyond time and history. I first heard about them during my stay at the Findhorn community in Scotland in 1977. St. Germain, who had a close relationship with several Findhorn members, was referred to often and described as being a master teacher from the White Brotherhood. I was also told that the Order of the Melchizedek was a part of the Brotherhood, and it is from this group that all of the major religious leaders come who have been a part of our history. As I have said, I ignored the Brotherhood and its existence for years, assuming that they knew how to do their job, whatever that was, very well without me and that my focus was primarily on nature, not on human-oriented evolution. After all, this is the age of specialization.

My understanding of how the Brotherhood functions is, I'm sure, somewhat simplistic. I see them operating in a co-creative role with us on this planet. They design and infuse purpose and direction into the frameworks of social order through which we on Earth move in order to learn, experience, and evolve. In essence, they create the schools through which we move. We call these schools religions, governmental structures, educational movements, philosophy, science... all those massive

4

social frameworks with which we associate and within which we function.

Let me say something about the name "White Brotherhood." Since publishing *MAP* in 1990, several people have written me questioning—and sometimes complaining about—that name. They want to make sure this isn't some white supremacist/sexist organization before buying *MAP* and getting into the program. Trust me, the White Brotherhood is neither. It includes males, females, and souls beyond both persuasions, and they can outdo us any day when it comes to color.

The name "White Brotherhood" has been used for this group for centuries. We did not coin the name here at Perelandra. It was coined by those folks on the Earth level who first began to consciously work with this group. It is not a name the group chose for itself. It is a name *we* chose for it. The words "white brotherhood" maintained the intent and integrity of the group, so it has always been acceptable to them. "White" is used to signify *all* the rays of the light spectrum. "Brotherhood" is used to signify not only the family of all *people* but also the family of all *life*.

If the name sticks in your throat and causes you a problem in deciding whether or not you would like to participate in MAP, here's what I suggest. Put aside your objections temporarily. Start the program and allow yourself enough time to get comfortably settled in. This should take four to six weeks, at most. Once you are settled, address your objections to the name "White

Brotherhood." If you still have objections, consider what name you would feel comfortable with that would maintain the intent of this vast group. Ask your MAP team if your name is acceptable to use when you are referring to this group. Unless you are way off base with your name, I'm sure they will have no objections. They will just need to know that when *you* say "Purple Peoplehood" or "Neutral Androgenyhood," you mean them.

One other point: Your special name for the White Brotherhood is between you and them. It would be neither helpful nor accurate to feel your name is for everyone and announce it to others. Not all of us have a problem with the name nor do we seek to change it. It would be more helpful to allow others to make their own decisions and work on their own with their team around this issue.

NATURE

As I mentioned earlier, my work with the White Brotherhood focuses on nature. The Medical Assistance Program (MAP) is an example of the Brotherhood and nature working together for our benefit within an organized framework that we call MAP: The Co-Creative White Brotherhood Medical Assistance Program.

The keystone of MAP is its coning. It is set up to assure perfect balance between the involution dynamic (nature) and the evolution dynamic (the White Brotherhood and you). The evolution dynamic supplies the purpose and definition to any thing or action. The involution dynamic (nature) supplies the matter, means, and action for achieving evolution's purpose and definition. The human soul is the force behind the evolution dynamic. Nature is the force behind involution. In health, the evolution dynamic comes from one's soul. It is from our soul that we receive the impulses that define our direction and purpose. It is the soul that gives the necessary data to nature for all that is physically required for a human to fully operate within a given lifetime. Nature then supplies us our body according to these soul-directed specifications. This also means that nature is the engineer of the human body and, like any good engineer, knows how it is supposed to work and how to fix it if it isn't working correctly.

In MAP, nature also anchors the program and makes it accessible to everyone on our level as well as to the medical teams in the White Brotherhood. Because of nature, we need not have an intermediary third party bridging us into the White Brotherhood. Nature's presence allows the medical teams to work with us directly.

Now, there are some fine books written about nature intelligences, how to communicate with them and how to work with them. I know this because I wrote some of them! I may not have been familiar with the White Brotherhood when MAP was begun, but I was sure familiar with nature. I don't want to bog you down with a boatload of information about nature or conings. But, to help with your understanding, I have included several definitions in this section and a section in the

Appendices (Appendix A) on conings. If you wish to understand more about nature intelligences in general, I recommend the *Perelandra Garden Workbook: A Complete Guide to Gardening with Nature Intelligences.*

The following is a good working definintion of nature. In fact, it is what nature gave me when I asked it to define ten key terms it uses often in the Perelandra research and work. (The full paper on definitions by nature is reprinted in Appendix E.)

NATURE: *In the larger universe and beyond, on its many levels and dimensions, there are a number of groups of consciousnesses that, although equal in importance, are quite different in expression and function. . . . Together, they make up the full expression of the larger, total life picture. No one piece, no one expression, can be missing or the larger life picture on all its levels and dimensions will cease to exist. One such consciousness has been universally termed "nature." Because of what we are saying about the larger picture not existing without all of its parts, you may assume that nature as both a reality and a consciousness exists on all dimensions and all levels. It cannot be excluded.*

Each group of consciousnesses has what can be termed an area of expertise. As we said, all groups are equal in importance but express and function differently from one another. These different expressions and functions are vital to the overall balance of reality. A truly symbiotic relationship exists among the groups and is based on balance—universal balance. . . . Nature is a massive, intelligent consciousness group that expresses and functions within the many areas of involution—that is, moving soul-oriented consciousness into any dimension or level of form.

Nature is the conscious reality that supplies order, organization, and life vitality for this shift. Nature is the consciousness that is, for your working understanding, intimately linked with form. Nature is the consciousness that comprises all form on all levels and dimensions. It is form's order, organization, and life vitality. Nature is first and foremost a consciousness of equal importance with all other consciousnesses in the largest scheme of reality. It expresses and functions uniquely in that it comprises all form on all levels and dimensions and is responsible for and creates all of form's order, organization, and life vitality.

To assist you in understanding "nature," I include nature's definition of form, devas, and nature spirits.

FORM: *We consider reality to be in the form state when there is order, organization, and life vitality combined with a state of consciousness. . . .*

We do not consider form to be only that which is perceptible to the five senses. In fact, we see form from this perspective to be most limited, both in its life reality and in its ability to function. We see form from the perspective of the five senses to be useful only for the most basic and fundamental level of identification. From this perspective, there is very little relationship to the full understanding and knowledge of how a unit or form system functions.

9

All energy contains order, organization, and life vitality; therefore, all energy is form. . . .

On the planet Earth, the personality, character, emotional makeup, intellectual capacity, strong points, and gifts of a human are all form. They are that which gives order, organization, and life vitality to consciousness.

Order and organization are the physical structures that create a framework for form. In short, they define the walls. But we have included the dynamic of life vitality when we refer to form because one of the elements of form is action, and it is the life vitality that initiates and creates action.

DEVAS AND NATURE SPIRITS: *"Devas" and "nature spirits" are names used to identify two different expressions and functions within the nature consciousness. They are the two groups within the larger nature consciousness that interface with the human soul while in form. There are other groups, and they are differentiated from one another primarily by specific expression and function.*

To expand from our definition of form, it is the devic expression that fuses with consciousness to create order, organization, and life vitality. The devic expression as the architect designs the complex order, organization, and life vitality that will be needed by the soul consciousness while functioning within the scope or band of form. If the consciousness chooses to shift from one point of form to another point, thereby changing form function, it is the devic expression of nature that alters the order, organization, and life vitality accordingly. The devic expression designs and is the creation of the order, organization, and life vitality of form.

10

The nature spirit expression infuses the devic order, organization, and life vitality and adds to this the dynamic of function and working balance. To order, organization, and life vitality it brings movement and the bond that maintains the alignment of the devic form unit to the universal principles of balance while the consciousness is in form.

*To say that nature is the expert in areas of form and form principles barely scratches the surface of the true nature (pardon the pun) of nature's role in form. It is the expert of form, and it is form itself. A soul-oriented consciousness cannot exist on any level or dimension of form in any way without an **equal**, intimate, symbiotic relationship with the nature consciousness.*

For you to work with MAP, you will be working with the White Brotherhood plus two specific nature intelligences from two different levels: the devic and the nature spirit levels. As stated in the above definition, these two names, "deva" and "nature spirit," are used to identify two different expressions and functions within the nature consciousness. The specific nature intelligences you will be working with are the Deva of Healing and Pan.

THE DEVA OF HEALING: As part of the devic level, this intelligence functions as an architectural force and creates the physical structures found within all human healing. The order, organization, and life vitality of the human body—that is, the full physical structure and how it functions—fall within the domain of the Deva of Healing. Since MAP is focused on the health and balance of us humans, it is critical that the nature intelligence responsible for the physical process of healing the human body be included in the coning. With its presence, the White Brotherhood is assured that all healing processes within MAP maintain the integrity of natural law to its fullest.

PAN: Pan is the traditional name for the nature spirit who oversees and coordinates the full nature spirit level. I call Pan the CEO of the nature spirit level. The devic level *creates* all of the blueprints for form. The nature spirit level *implements* those blueprints—they are the builders. It also coordinates the action and movement of all form and ensures that this activity maintains the integrity of the original devic blueprint. In MAP, Pan aligns all physical elements of any action or process that might occur in a session to the devic healing blueprint.

We work with Pan in MAP because he is the only nature spirit that does not have regional limitations. He is universal in dynamic. This means that everyone, no matter where they are positioned on the planet, can work with Pan. His universality is critical for a program that was intended to be global. (By the way, Pan is actually without, or beyond, gender. I refer to him as "him" because his energy feels masculine to me during our communications.)

And finally, it is the nature spirit level, represented by Pan, that keys our physical presence into the medical units of the White Brotherhood and stabilizes that presence during the session.

Let me tell you a little about how this program came into existence. As I have mentioned, the expansion of my work with nature into this new level of teamwork with the Brotherhood required that I physically shift and operate in new ways that would support and process the new level of work. It was such a massive jump for me that my body systems did not know how to adjust to the new demands. The first thing that occurred was that I began to misalign structurally. I had worked with a chiropractor for years previous to this as part of my general maintenance health program, and I knew my body was structurally strong. I rarely needed a chiropractic adjustment. Now I needed them once or twice a month, and the adjustments were fairly extensive. At first, I said nothing to my chiropractor about the new level of work. But, after the first visit, she mentioned that something was odd. I was suddenly requiring a lot of adjustments and not requiring flower essences. (She routinely includes flower essence testing in her work.) Normally, when she sees the scope of adjustments I was needing, they are emotionally induced and require flower essences stabilization. I was not testing positive for the essences. Though she didn't voice them, she was beginning to have questions.

After the second visit, during which I required as many adjustments as the first, I told her briefly what I was doing and something about its effect on my work and life. She didn't even blink. She just said that explained what she was seeing. My body didn't know how to process what I was now working with and it was "flying out of alignment" from the strain. I would need periodic adjustments while my body system was learning how to function within the new level of reality.

The second major problem I had to face was the sudden development of head pain. I felt as if my head wanted to explode. It wasn't a conventional headache— it was more like somebody had an air hose hooked up to my head and was pumping in air well beyond the capacity that my head could hold.

I returned to the chiropractor and told her about the head pressure. Luckily, she is one of five percent of chiropractors in the United States who are trained in cranial adjustments. My physical system had to pick up the new impulses and translate them accurately in order to process what was happening to me, perceive accurately what I was working with, and function well within that perception. All this is accomplished primarily within the sacrum, spinal column, and cranials, and it directly impacts the flow and pulsations of the cerebrospinal fluid. It is also along the spinal column that impulses are first processed by the nervous system. We could see by the adjustments I needed that all of this new action was having an impact on my sacrum, spine, and head. The body, not knowing how to receive such a

14

massive infusion of impulses or how to translate this input accurately, reacted by either overloading or closing down. Physically, this would result in misalignment of the sacrum, vertebrae, and/or misalignment or jamming of the cranials. The skull is composed of ten major cranial bones that expand and contract according to the ebb and flow of the cerebrospinal fluid. The massive infusion of new impulses was akin to throwing a monkey wrench into this normal physical operation and knocking things out of kilter. Hence, the head pain.

My chiropractor and I worked together to assist my body in shifting to a different structural alignment that would better facilitate the new work I was doing. I could then learn how to process the new impulses with ease and accuracy. For a year and a half, we worked together. We responded to the glitches as they occurred (these were easy for me to detect since they resulted in various degrees of pain). The chiropractor was smart enough not to dictate what alignment I should be in; rather, she observed what alignment my body was moving toward and assisted that movement.

Our work was brought to a climax after a year and a half when my parietal cranials moved into what the chiropractor called a "parietal spread." These two massive bones at the top of the skull assumed a position allowing their expansion and contraction to operate within a new, expanded range. With this, the head pain was relieved. The chiropractor said she felt that all of our work over the past year and a half had led to this one major adjustment. We both felt that our work together had gone as far as it could go.

For a few months, all was well. But in the summer of 1984, the head pain returned. I remember I was in the garden when I realized that my head was beginning to hurt. I guess, as is often the case in these moments of change, I felt my work with the chiropractor was no longer feasible for practical reasons. Her office is an hour and a half drive from Perelandra, and her practice is so large that I often had to wait a week or two for an appointment. For some reason, none of this had made any difference to me when I went to her previously. But now it was unacceptable. I felt I could not wait to have this head pain alleviated, and I was unwilling to continue driving such a long distance for what I now thought would be never-ending treatment.

A thought popped into my mind. Perhaps the White Brotherhood could somehow be of assistance. With my head pain increasing, I figured it was worth a shot. I connected with the White Brotherhood, told them my problem, and asked if there was something they could do to help me. They told me to go lie down, open a coning (this will be explained later), and they would connect me with help. I followed their instructions—and met Lorpuris, the head of the White Brotherhood Medical Unit.

I explained to Lorpuris what my physical discomforts were and tried to describe them as fully as I could. He instructed me to just lie quietly and comfortably, and he then set to work. The session lasted about an hour, during which I felt as if I was getting an energy charge or current through different parts of my body. It wasn't painful at all, but I must admit that it was so different from anything I had ever felt that I found the sensations to be both exciting and a little scary. At the end of the hour, Lorpuris suggested that we meet regularly so that I could go through comprehensive body balancing to facilitate my new level of operation. I agreed and we "made a date." When I closed down the session and walked back outside, I realized that my head no longer hurt. I was amazed.

Since 1984, Lorpuris and I have continued to meet regularly. In the process of helping me physically and emotionally to adjust to my ever-expanding work and life, we explored various ways in which he and his extensive medical unit could work with others here on Earth in areas of health and healing. In fact, they had been interested in making this kind of connection with us for some time.

But there were two major problems that had to be surmounted in order for us to successfully work with the White Brotherhood Medical Unit. First, there was the problem of their keying into our life system on all levels (physical, emotional, mental, and spiritual) and maintaining that connection with us clearly and long enough for a medical session. We solved this problem by bringing nature on board as a member of the Brotherhood team. When I connect with my medical team, I do it within a coning, a vortex of energy that includes nature intelligences, the medical team, and me. Within this coning vortex, nature is able to stabilize us on all levels with the Brotherhood.

The second problem involved communication between us and our medical team. They did not want to establish a working relationship that would exclude all but the few who knew how to receive interlevel communication. We solved this problem in two ways. The MAP sessions have built into them schedules and time frames that enable everyone to utilize the program even if they are unable to sense or hear anything from their team. All people have to do is follow the MAP instructions and the schedule. They don't have to hear from their team when they should meet with them or for how long. This is already spelled out for them. All they have to do is talk—tell the team what is going on with them and what is out of sorts. The team can hear us effortlessly even if we can't hear them. The other solution to the communication problem was kinesiology. Those who want to ask questions and receive answers from their team can do so by using a simple yes/no format. Then, they can "read" the answers from their team by kinesiology testing. This opens the communication door from both sides. (See Appendix B for how to do kinesiology.)

Another point about communication: When we first enter MAP, we may not be able to hear or sense our team. (But we will sense things happening to us physically from time to time during the sessions.) As we continue the program, we will become used to our team, be better able to process the input from them, and we will have gone through some of the clearing and adjustments necessary for us to hear and sense our team, and not just experience their work.

We have cleared up these two major stumbling blocks, and as a result MAP was created. The shingle has been hung. The office is now open. And you are invited to enter the program.

Chapter 2

How MAP
Can Help You

To give you an idea of how MAP came into my life, I have talked about a somewhat exceptional development that most people would not encounter in their lives, but that was responsible for leading me into MAP. However, I don't want to leave the impression that MAP is only for exceptional times It is not. MAP is for those who feel that their present medical support—whether traditional or alternative—is not enough. For years, you may have felt absolutely comfortable with your medical support, and then suddenly, without a shadow of a doubt, you know you need more. To function *well* you need more input, more support. Yet, when you look around and try alternatives, none feel right. MAP is then your answer.

Because the MAP team includes nature, MAP is a *physical* program (not a spiritual program) that works on your well-being from the physical, emotional, mental, and spiritual perspective. And because of the unique position of the MAP team, it works on strains, pressures, pain, and conflict being felt on all these levels

21

simultaneously. When it comes to health issues, these four levels interrelate. Normally we go to professionals who are experts in one level or one area of a level. It is up to us to put a team together that addresses the different aspects of the problem. And, when we put these teams together, they rarely consult with one another. So we don't have a sense of a united and coordinated medical approach. The MAP teams work on all levels simultaneously and function as a coordinated unit. Consequently, a MAP session is more comprehensive and its results are deeper than those of other health systems.

We can initiate MAP during times of illness and injury, or it can be initiated during times of relative health when we feel we are capable of a better level of health and balance—and we want it. MAP is a comprehensive health program that you will use throughout your entire life. It is not a one-time program only for emergency situations. We are constantly changing and developing throughout our lives. MAP helps us maintain a high level of balance and function throughout all our changes and shifts. In short, it gives us a chance to experience an exceptional quality of life.

We can begin MAP at any stage in our life and at any age. We do not have to be healthy to begin (some have thought this was necessary!), and we do not have to be sick. We do not need to abandon any medical support we have been using in order to begin MAP. If you are combining other health practices with MAP, this is fine. Just tell your MAP team what other things you are involved in and how. MAP will accommodate them. As I worked with my team and experienced the depth of their work, I gradually dropped the other health practices I had been using, one by one. My confidence about MAP had to grow before I felt comfortable switching my medical needs to MAP exclusively. However, if I had a serious illness or injury that common sense told me needed quick medical attention, I would not hesitate to get it. The difference is that I would work with my MAP team throughout the problem, as well.

It is important that you understand one thing about working with a White Brotherhood MAP team. *They will not, under any circumstances, circumvent your timing on any issue.* You are in complete control and command of your timing and rate of development. They will not circumvent your timing, because it would be wrong to do so. This would, in effect, remove you from the driver's seat in your own life and place you in the position of a child being catered to by the almighty parent. Your team will simply not participate in such activity.

In MAP, *you* control your timing and development in an interesting way. You will note in the instructions that you are urged to talk to your team. Tell them everything that comes to mind that is bothering you on any of your PEMS levels (physical, emotional, mental, and spiritual). You aren't going through this exercise because your team is stupid and can't see you are in trouble. The troubles or situations you can articulate to your team tell them what you are ready to work on. And the extent to which you can describe the situation tells them the extent to which you are ready to change what is bothering

23

you. *You are your own barometer.* They will not work in areas beyond those you recognize and describe. Consequently, your team will never put you in a position of facing and dealing with something for which you are unprepared. In the MAP sessions, *you* are your own master, and your team assists you in achieving your goals of health and balance in ways that are beyond belief. You are simply demonstrating your wisdom by choosing the best team with which to work.

SESSION: LORPURIS

I would like to add a bit to what Machaelle has already written. In short, I would like to assure you that we are eager to assist you in your quest for health and balance in any way you see fit. There will be those who will gravitate to MAP and wish to establish themselves in the program, but they will hesitate because they will feel unworthy of such an expanded approach or feel inferior, believing that we would consider it bothersome to work with them. It is this situation I would like to address.

I would like to point out that it is not a sign of good health and balance if individuals refuse help despite the fact they have gravitated toward the very help they are refusing. You might feel that I am stating the obvious. But we see the greatest stumbling block in establishing the kind of medical assistance that so many are presently seeking, either consciously or unconsciously, as being this issue of feeling unworthy of the help. It is a vicious cycle—and one we cannot step in from "out of the blue" and release a person from.

24

*We suggest that if the concept of MAP feels right to you, yet you are feeling hesitant because you can't believe something "so good" could come to you, that you temporarily put aside your hesitancies for the purpose of entering the program. As we have said, feeling unworthy—and I use the word "unworthy" to cover feelings such as inferiority, weakness, fear, and lack of capability—is a sign of being in need of help. Once you have entered the program **and have discussed with us the reasons for your hesitancies,** we will then be able to work with you to obtain a new level of balance that will effectively adjust your sense of self-worth and thus take care of the very reason you might not have entered the program.*

In the MAP workshops I have given at Perelandra, this issue of self worth has come up often. Invariably, someone will say he or she simply can't understand why a medical team from the White Brotherhood would choose to work with them. And, if the White Brotherhood does this kind of work with them, doesn't it mean that they are being chosen by the Brotherhood to then do something significant—like save the world or something? Surely you can't remain "just a housewife" or a car mechanic if you have a MAP team.

In the overall picture, the White Brotherhood is presently focused on shifting all that exists on this planet from a Piscean dynamic (parent/child) to an Aquarian dynamic (teamwork). Everything must shift. And all of us are involved in this shift. No one is exempt. We are responsible for catching on to what's happening and doing the work needed to make this shift. The MAP medical teams are not doing something extraordinary for a handful of "chosen" people. This program is for everyone who wants it. By working with us individually, the MAP teams assist us in living life with a better balance and getting on with the changes that are needed. Everything that is involved in the work of a housewife or auto mechanic must go through this shift, as well. The last thing a MAP team wants you to do is throw away everything and go off to "save the world." MAP wants you to do what you are meant to do, do it the best you can, and take responsibility for shifting your piece of the life puzzle from the Piscean picture to the Aquarian picture. It's all important to MAP. No one is insignificant.

EXPANDED EXPERIENCES AND MAP

Since the MAP program developed as a response to my struggles with integrating an expanded level of operation, I asked Lorpuris to explain how we operate during times of expansion.

Now, don't get confused here. MAP is for general health balance, regular health issues, extraordinary health issues, and assistance during expansion experiences. It's not only for expansion experiences. But I find that people often reach the point of feeling that they need more from their medical support system because of the physical and emotional pressure that expansion experiences place on them. Expansion experiences have traditionally been relegated to spirituality, and many feel that only those who are "spiritually evolved" have expansion experiences. Well, this simply isn't true. We all have expansion experiences. Any time we learn something new, that's expansion. Any time we experience something new, that, too, is expansion. Whatever is new to us must be received and processed accurately and well in order for the experience to be useful.

I have said that a good sign a person needs MAP is when he has a deep sense that he needs more medical support than is presently available to him. Many feel the need for additional help when struggling with especially challenging expansion experiences because, as a rule, traditional and alternative medical systems prevalent today do not accept or understand that the human body plays an essential role during expansion. They don't understand or accept how the body functions at these times or what help we need if we are not functioning well. The next session will be helpful to those of you who recognize that you have been backed into a corner because of difficulties arising from expansion.

In explaining to me the role of the body in expansion, Lorpuris also gave a good explanation of how we operate as body/soul life systems on our planet. I think this will be helpful, in general, in understanding why we would feel the need for new medical assistance.

LORPURIS: HOW WE PHYSICALLY
SUPPORT EXPANSION

An expanded experience does not by definition mean it to be nonphysical or beyond five-senses form. It simply implies that the experience is beyond that which the person has experienced prior to that time—thus, the sense of expansion. We have said to you that the band of form is quite complex, and this is true. It includes all that a person can potentially experience while participating within any given level of form such as Earth.

While participating within a level of form such as Earth, all reality adheres to the universal law of horizontal compatibility. Consequently, what is expressed within the Earth level is "of form" whether it be discernible to the naked eye or not. The limitation regarding form arises when an individual defines form strictly from the perspective of the five senses. Nature, for example, does not distinguish between the tree as seen by the naked eye and the nature spirit of the tree that is not seen. To nature, both are fully "of form" and, therefore, have impact on and respond to one another within the laws of form.

Now, the laws of form are much broader than what is encompassed when one thinks of the five-senses sensory system. In fact, an expanded experience is simply learning or allowing the sensory system, as most individuals know it, to operate in a fuller capacity. The problem is that individuals see the five-senses system as the one and only sensory system, and anything beyond or outside this base functioning as being something entirely different. In fact, they are both functions of the same system.

When a child is born into the Earth level, its sensory system is quite sensitive and expanded. It is, after all, just moving from a state of being prior to birth in which the sensory system naturally functions in a broader state. If left on its own, the child would continue to develop its sensory system from the point of this broader perspective. And what one might call "expanded experiences" would be the norm. Societal preconceptions are what encourage the child to limit the sensory scope, and the development of the sensory system throughout childhood then takes place from this more limited perspective. Along with this, the limited definition of the sensory system and its scope of discernment becomes the rule of thumb by which to judge experience.

Now, if the sensory system is capable of naturally operating in a much broader scope than most individuals can at present imagine, it follows that the physical body must respond to and support that operation. The sensory system itself is a part of that overall body response and support system. Everything works as a team, ideally. Consequently, one cannot have what is known as an expanded experience without the sensory system and the physical body system as a whole responding to and attempting to support it. So, one may see a meditative state as an expanded experience, but, in fact, it is a broader use of the sensory system and draws appropriate response and support from within the physical body itself. Just as one cannot move a finger or toe without the entire body's muscular and skeletal systems responding, one cannot shift from one state of mind to another without a similar physical response and shift.

There is a saying many on the Earth level use: "If you don't

*use it, you lose it." Normally, this refers to muscle and body
tone. When a child limits the scope of operation within the
sensory system, the complementary scope of physical response
and support is no longer needed or utilized. In those areas, a
person stiffens and atrophies. Then, later on, when the individual is an adult and consciously chooses to reactivate the
sensory system in a broader way, the physical body no longer
"knows" how to respond and support that expansion. The person will experience nothing, no matter how much willpower
he musters, or the experience will be partially perceived and
most likely distorted, as well.*

*Let's address the body system itself and what happens when
the sensory system responds to an experience. Any experience
initially strikes the human body through the electrical system.
This occurs whether the experience is easily perceived or not.
The initial receptor of experience is not the brain or the senses
but the electrical system. The impact immediately, almost
simultaneously, shifts and translates into the nervous system
and routes itself throughout the nervous system appropriately
as it begins its identification and experience process. This includes activating the sensory system in an appropriate manner. (All this occurs within a split second.) The point to
remember is that the initial level of impact is electrical, followed by an impact on the nervous system. If the experience is
within the individual's perceived notion of "acceptable," this
usually means that the person knows how to perceive the experience on all levels operating within the physical body.*

*Two things can occur if the individual doesn't know what to
do with the experience. Either the physical body doesn't know*

how to respond and support the experience and is in need of assistance, or the experience itself is so beyond the person's operating scope of reality that it takes on an intensification that literally overwhelms the body and requires of it a level of operation well beyond its present range of capability.

In the latter case, the person must have a good foundation for such a stretch, or else he risks damaging himself physically. You would not want a person who is not capable of walking a half-mile to suddenly be forced to run three miles. But you could expect someone who easily runs three miles could tackle a seven-mile run without sustaining damage. It's a challenge, but it is not beyond the scope of possibility, and most likely not dangerous. However, the body used to the exertion of the three-mile run would have a challenge with responding well to the longer run, and it could result in soreness and discomfort until the body learns to support the longer run.

Addressing the case of your 1982 expansion, Machaelle: You had the foundation for the challenge. You could run the three miles with ease and grace. This we were sure of. The question was how you were going to process the intensity of the new input. All that occurred was initially received within the electrical system and then shifted into the nervous system. In some ways, you responded physically much more quickly than we anticipated. In other instances, the experience overwhelmed your system and assistance was needed. Note in the work done on you by the chiropractor that she maintained close proximity to the electrical and nervous systems by concentrating her work on the spine, sacrum, and cranials.

Let me sum up the relationship of the cranial/spine/sacrum

31

with the expanded experience. *The experience is received electrically, shifted to the nervous system for sorting and identification, and, at this point, the physical body systems move to support what is being identified. If the body cannot adequately shift, the electrical system will overload or break, and the corresponding vertebrae, sacrum, or cranials will most likely react by misaligning. Hence you have the sensation of trying to catch six balls all at once while only being able to catch four.*

A SPECIAL NOTE ABOUT THE CRANIALS: An expanded experience carries with it an intensity that registers through the electrical system, moves into the nervous system, and continues its impact into the cerebrospinal fluid. The brain is impacted by both the nervous system activity and the CSF (cerebrospinal fluid) pulse response to the impact. The cranial plates must respond accordingly to accommodate this two-pronged impact. The range of plate movement will be affected. If the cranials have lost their knowledge of how to move within this new range or if they are three-milers stretching for the seven-mile run, they run the risk of jamming or misaligning. This is when so much of the head pain associated with expanded experience comes up. Cranial adjustments may be necessary over a period of time in order to allow time for the plates to properly adjust to and move in a more expanded range. One may receive these adjustments either from a physician such as a chiropractor or from MAP.

Just as the leg muscles need to adjust to the seven-mile run, the cranials need time to adjust to expansion. Because of the close working proximity with the electrical and nervous systems, the cranials must be considered one of the primary areas for assistance during times of expansion. In a relatively short period of time, the cranials, as well as the rest of the physical body system, will learn how to operate within the expanded range of experience with ease, accuracy, and efficiency.

Chapter 3

How to Work
with MAP

Read through this chapter in its entirety before doing your first MAP session. It will give you a good foundation. There are quick-reference steps in Chapter 8 that you can use when doing a session.

THE FIRST SESSION

Lie down. Get comfortable. You will need to lie on your back and remain in that position during the entire session, which lasts one hour. *Also, while lying down, do not cross your legs or your hands and arms over your body.* NOTE: If you have to do or get something during the session that requires that you cross your arms over your body, that's fine. When you're finished, just remember to put your arms back along your sides. Also, you might wish to cover yourself with a blanket, even a thin blanket in the summer. Besides keeping you warm, it may make you feel more secure. If you have back pain or are having trouble getting comfortable, try placing a pillow under your knees. If sitting in a comfortable chair

35

makes it easier for you to remain alert and relaxed, then do it. In short, do what you need to do in order to remain alert and be comfortable.

By the way, the MAP team does not care if you are wearing clothes—or, in other words, they don't require that you get naked! You can wear a belt, polyester, naturally dyed garments or unnaturally dyed garments. What you are wearing is not an issue to the MAP teams. The only criteria is that you are comfortable.

1. Open the MAP coning. (Relax! Keep reading. "Coning" gets explained.)

> Overlighting Deva of Healing
> Pan
> White Brotherhood Medical Unit
> Your higher self

To open this coning, state (aloud or to yourself): I would like to open a MAP coning. I would like to be connected with the following:

> Overlighting Deva of Healing—Either wait ten seconds for the connection or use kinesiology (explained in Appendix B) to verify the connection.
>
> Pan—Wait ten seconds or verify.
>
> White Brotherhood Medical Unit—Wait ten seconds or verify.
>
> My higher self—Wait ten seconds or verify.

Wait another ten to fifteen seconds to adjust to the coning.

The coning is now open and you are ready to begin.

It's that simple. It is not important if you did not have any sensations as the coning was activated. Your sensations or lack of sensations will not affect the quality of the coning in any way. What is important is that you be the one to call the coning into activation.

ABOUT CONINGS: Since the 1990 publication of *MAP*, people have expressed interest in knowing more about a coning—what it is, what it does, and how it works. You don't have to understand a coning in order to open a MAP coning. All you have to do is go through step 1 and the coning automatically opens. Then you can proceed with the session. If you want to know more about conings, turn to Appendix A. If this coning business doesn't interest you right now, just go on to step 2.

2. The first session will be for scanning purposes only. This is the one session when you need not talk to your team if you don't wish. The purpose of this session is to key you into their level, identify your various energy patterns, lock in your life systems on all PEMS levels, and get the appropriate medical team identified and working with you. This team will work with you during all your medical sessions. Occasionally, when the situation calls for it, another member of the medical unit will join your team to lend expertise for a special situation. In these instances, the team will expand on its own to include whoever is necessary. You do not have to do anything special for this to occur. Your primary team will be those who work with you during the majority of your sessions.

The scanning session will last an hour. You may feel gentle shifts and energy flowing throughout your body during this session. Or you may even feel like you are floating or moving. You also may feel absolutely nothing. Don't worry about this. The work is going on. You might want to set a timer or alarm for one hour when you begin the session so that if you should drift or fall asleep, you'll know when the session is over and when to go on to step 3.

3. At the end of the hour, request that you be given your code—a symbol, word, or sensation that you can use to identify your team. *Whatever pops into your mind next will be it.* Don't discount what happens once you request the code. When opening a coning for any future medical sessions, add this identification (visualize or speak it) when you call the White Brotherhood Medical Unit into the coning. This will link you more efficiently with your team. Another way of saying this is: The code is the "extension number" you will use when connecting with your MAP team. It allows you to bypass the White Brotherhood "main switchboard." It might be good to write or draw your symbol right after this first session just to make sure you recall it accurately later on.

Many have gotten nervous when they get to this part of the process because they feel they won't be able to discern their team identification or code. In fact, some use this as an excuse not to do MAP. Well, all I can say is that you've got to try this to believe it. Many people who swore they could never be "sensitive" enough to get their code have gathered in their courage and asked the question. Lo and behold, up pops their code. They hear a word or a phrase, or they visualize a scene, or suddenly recall a special scene from their past, or see colors, or hear sounds, or feel a strong, clear sensation. Whatever it is, that's their team identification.

Your team identification can be fun. They can sound like something out of the CIA code book: Torch, Lancer, Deep Rest, NIMO, Bunny-Love, Crystal Dove, or, my personal favorite, I Gotta Pee. . . . Other people get visual symbols: the peace symbol, trees, a specific flower, clasped hands, the sun, shafts of light. . . . And still others see color. When they open the coning, they identify their team by visualizing or looking at a specific color.

These identifiers don't have to be wrought with deep esoteric meaning; they just have to be something that you and your team agree upon. And they're not secret. You don't compromise MAP or your team in any way if you share what your code is with others. And no one else can use your code. Someone else may have a code name that is similar, even the same as yours, but when that code is linked with you/your energy field, as it is when you are opening a MAP coning, it becomes unique to you, and you automatically connect with your team.

Also, I have heard from some folks who, after working with MAP for a while, wanted to change their identifying code or symbol. Sometimes they just sense the name should be changed, or they feel that their team now has permanent new members. You can either request a new code from your team or suggest one yourself. What's important is that your team is very clear about the new identification. Or, you'll be in a session, not sensing that any change is needed, when a new code suddenly pops into mind. However the new code is derived, describe it fully to the team during that MAP session. Most likely, they will either flash the new symbol or "sound" the new code back to you to indicate their code for you has now changed. Or you can kinesiology test that it is acceptable with the team.

If you don't hear or sense a code during this first session, relax. You can continue with MAP without a code. For future sessions, just continue to set up the coning as you did for this scanning session. You will then be connected with your team. It's like you call into the main switchboard and then your call gets transferred to the right party. As mentioned above, using the symbol makes this process more efficient. But not using a symbol doesn't prevent your having a MAP session. Eventually, you will "receive" the code.

4. At the end of the hour, close the coning. You do this by focusing on each member of the coning separately, thanking that member, and asking to be disconnected. A coning closes as easily as it opens. You need do nothing fancy. If you use kinesiology, verify that you are disconnected from each member by asking, "Am I disconnected?" (Test.) You'll get a "yes." If you don't, it means you weren't focused when you requested that the

coning be closed. Collect yourself and do step 4 over. This time when you test to verify, it will be closed.

If you are using flower essences, do a basic test and check to see if you need a dosage. These essences will help stabilize you after your first experience in a MAP coning. However, if you are not using flower essences, you'll be fine. Spend a few moments quietly before going on about your day. Bouncing out of a MAP session could feel like a jolt. (See Appendix C for flower essence testing steps.)

Wait twenty-four hours before opening the next session. The body needs twenty-four hours to adjust to the impact of the coning and the expansion of working with the White Brotherhood team. Once you have waited the twenty-four hours and you have done your first regular session, you need not wait twenty-four hours again before opening MAP. If you are sick, you may wish to open MAP daily or even twice a day for assistance as you move through the illness.

REGULAR MAP SESSION PROCESS

If you use flower essences, place them within easy reach. If you do not use flower essences or have never heard of them, I highly recommend that you investigate them and consider adding them to your health program. Having experienced MAP since 1984, I can say that flower essences are a tremendous help. Also, the MAP teams prefer you to use the essences as well. They are used in conjunction with the MAP sessions to stabilize us after the session and assist in our integrating the work the MAP team has done. There are times when the work will take, if left on its own, twenty-four hours to shift into and complete its impact on the physical body. Flower essences make these shifts efficient, effortless, and complete within a two-hour period at the most. I have included information on flower essences in Appendix C. The flower essence testing instructions that are given in the steps will be understood by those who use flower essences. But again, if you do not have flower essences and don't wish to include them, this does not stop you from participating fully in MAP.

Lie down on your back or sit. Get comfortable. Cover yourself with a blanket if you wish.

1. Open the MAP coning. Wait ten seconds after each connection.

Overlighting Deva of Healing
Pan
Your White Brotherhood Medical Team—Visualize your team's symbol or say the code word.
Your higher self

Wait ten to fifteen seconds after activating the full coning so that your body can stabilize itself within the coning and with the team.

2. If they are available, test yourself for flower essences. Take the essences that you test are needed. Do not bother testing for dosage since you will be testing again

after the session is complete. If you are not using essences, skip this step.

3. Focus your attention on the session and your team. If you can't feel or sense your team, just keep your focus on the session. Describe *as fully as you can* how you are feeling. This includes how you feel physically, emotionally, mentally, and spiritually. Relax about what you are not able to articulate. You get better with practice. (*Remember: This step is crucial for indicating your personal timing and rhythm. Your team will never alter or bypass your timing and rhythm. What you can articulate, you are ready to address.*)

This is where people begin to feel like hypochondriacs or that they are pestering their team with "silly little things" that aren't really a problem.

Let me say something about symptoms that might help get you over this hurdle. Symptoms create a crucial, active communication between you and your body when you are not functioning in balance. They become an effective tool when we are working with a medical team that understands the full ramification of each symptom and knows what to do with them.

In the medical world, symptoms are used for achieving an overall definition or label from which a doctor can choose a prescribed course of action, which is then superimposed onto the symptoms.

With MAP, symptoms are important tools for determining complexity, degree, rhythm, and timing.

When describing symptoms to your team, be precise—

43

or as precise as you can be. Don't just say you feel emotional when you could break it down by saying you feel teary eyed, vulnerable, and easily irritated when people say certain things to you. (Then describe those things.) Don't just say you have a headache when you could be more specific by saying you have pain and pressure in the upper right side of your left eye and across the middle of your forehead. And learn the differences between an ache, a pain, and a shooting pain.

Remember, symptoms are the communication between you and your body. By accurately describing them to your team, they become the communication between you and your team, as well. The symptoms you are able to perceive and how accurately you are able to describe them tells your team precisely what you are ready to work on.

As I've said, your team isn't stupid. They know what your imbalances are. By describing how you are feeling to your team, you are telling them which of the imbalances you are ready to work with.

CAUTION: Some people have tried to get around this issue of talking to their team about symptoms by just giving the team a blanket invitation to work on everything—now. This is foolhardy, and your team will not accept the invitation. It would be risky to your health and well-being if you were moved from an imbalanced state to one of balance all at one time.

Also, quite a few people diagnose their own symptoms. They're doing exactly what doctors do. I must admit that in a lot of cases, their guess is as good as the doctor's. They look at the collection of symptoms, then figure out what illness or disease these symptoms best describe. But I recommend that, when working with MAP, you do not self-diagnose. Just describe the symptoms. For example, don't say, "I have shingles." You might not have shingles, but apparently you know what constitutes shingles. Your mental label could get in the way of what is really going on with you, and although your team already knows you don't have shingles, what's important in this situation is what *you think* you have. You may have unwittingly created a block that has complicated your true illness, which can't be eliminated until you discard the self-diagnosis.

4. Allow forty minutes for the session to be completed. If you feel uncomfortable during the session, tell your team what you are feeling (this includes physical and emotional discomfort), and then relax and trust that at the end, whatever adjustments and shifts that were making you uncomfortable will have been completed.

If flower essences are available, ask your team during uncomfortable times if you need to test for them. If you can't actually "hear" your team, use kinesiology to get their answer. If you test positive, simply test the essences and take the ones you need (do not get dosage information), and then resume the session. The team will wait while you test. Also, if you should get an intuitive hit to test essences, either check with your team and ask if they want you to test (if you can directly communicate with them), or assume your intuition is correct and test.

However, before testing essences, tell your team you feel the need to do so. They will hold up their work while you do this. If your intuition was wrong, you'll just test that you need no essences. It's certainly worth checking out, and your team does not mind if you do so.

It's important that you move around as little as possible during a session, so you will need to have the essences beside you for testing. Now, you don't have to get crazy with this. What I mean is that it's better to have the essence boxes available beside you during a session than to leave them downstairs in the kitchen and have to get them during a session. Also, if you change your position or need to go to the bathroom during a session, tell your team to hold it a minute, do what is needed as quickly as possible, lie down again, and return to the session.

Sometimes their work will make you feel like you want to curl up in a fetal position. Don't do it. Just remain on your back and tell your team about this urge. Shortly the team will have moved you through the process or cycle so that you will no longer feel the need to curl up.

Another point: Don't be afraid to talk to your team during a session. It is especially helpful if you give them a running commentary of what sensations you are feeling, if any, so they can read on the spot how you are processing the work they are doing. If you suddenly feel pain, let them know where it is and how intense it is. Your body is working very hard on all of its levels to make shifts and changes. Sometimes, something gets a

little "hung up" in the process. That's why your feedback is so important. (They are also open to hearing any
good jokes you might have as they work.)

Some people have said they feel a little odd talking to
their team. After all, no one but you is visible in the
room. They fear that anyone overhearing them may
think they've tripped around the loony bend. It *is* helpful to speak out loud. Your team doesn't care; they can
"hear" you if you say it out loud or silently. But it is
helpful to you. When we speak out loud, it is easier—
much easier—to maintain our focus on what we're
saying. This is important if we are a little tired going
into a session and intend to stay awake. So, I recommend that you say it out loud—but, you don't have to
shout it! Just say it softly. Make sure you can hear yourself while, at the same time, no one in the next room can
hear you.

5. At the end of forty minutes (add a few minutes for
opening the coning, essence testing, disruptions, or
bathroom timeouts you may have taken during the session), thank your team and close the session by dismantling the coning.

Dismantling the coning is as easy as activating it. State
(aloud or to yourself): I'd like to close the coning. I'd
like to disconnect from:

> Overlighting Deva of Healing
>
> Pan
>
> My White Brotherhood Medical Team
>
> My higher self

Wait ten to fifteen seconds for the dismantling to fully occur, or kinesiology test to verify that the coning is now closed.

6. Test yourself for flower essences. This time get the dosage (number of days and number of times per day you are to take the essence solution). This essence solution is what you need to stabilize the MAP work for you. Begin your dosage immediately after closing down the session. You may wish to spend a few minutes quietly before continuing with your day.

NOTE: If your essence dosage period extends into your next MAP session, discontinue that dosage after that session and test for new essences and a new dosage. Each MAP session will wipe the essence "slate" clean and will begin a new solution of essences and dosage.

MAP Session Schedule

IF YOU HAVE NO SERIOUS ILLNESS, DISEASE, OR INJURY: The following schedule is how the team would like to work with you for the first five months. This schedule applies to those of you who can communicate directly with your team and those of you who cannot. After working with thousands of people in MAP since 1990, the teams prefer this beginning schedule for those of you who do not have a serious, pre-existing illness, disease, or injury.

After five months, the teams recommend that sessions be held monthly for balancing and general maintenance.

However, if a specific difficulty, illness, or injury should arise *during or after* this five-month period, have MAP sessions twice weekly while going through these periods. If you sense more is needed to get you through the rough time, have sessions three to four times weekly. Once you are through this period, go back to where you were in the rhythm before the problem arose.

The beginning schedule:

First month — twice weekly

Second through fourth months — once weekly

Fifth month — monthly (for balancing and general maintenance)

During times of difficulty, illness, or while going through periods of challenging expansion — twice weekly If you sense more is needed: three or four times weekly.

Once you can communicate with your team, either through kinesiology or intuitive input, after the five-month beginning schedule, you can ask for specific guidelines for the schedule that are geared to your personal needs. Or you can just remain on the monthly schedule until a specific need arises. Then have MAP sessions two, three, or four times weekly, depending on what you sense is needed.

FOR THOSE ENTERING MAP WITH SERIOUS ILLNESS, INJURY, OR DISEASE: The MAP teams request the following schedule:

First month — twice weekly

Second through fifth month — once weekly
Continue on the weekly schedule until you have
moved through the illness, injury, or disease.

After the fifth month, assuming you can communicate
with your team, you may ask for specific guidelines for
the schedule that are geared to your needs. If you cannot
get this information, assume you are to stay on the
weekly schedule if you are still moving through the illness, injury, or disease.

Once you have completed the fifth month *and* you
have completely moved through the serious problem,
have MAP sessions twice a month for the next two
months. After this, have a session monthly for balancing
and general maintenance.

During times of difficulty, illness, or while going
through challenging periods of expansion, go back to
having sessions twice weekly. If you sense more is
needed, have them three or four times weekly.

Finding the Time to Do MAP

You've just gotten depressed because you don't know
how in the world you are going to keep up with this
schedule. Many people who have started MAP have
faced this problem. A number of mothers of small
children have told me that they actually get someone to
babysit the kids during their MAP sessions. Others have
said they play mind tricks on themselves—and they
work! They say they pretend the MAP sessions are a

class, or a doctor's appointment, or a racquetball game, or a meeting—something that requires them to literally carve out the time and create the schedule for it. To just have something to do at home doesn't give them enough of a reason to make the time. So they pretend it is one of those things that would normally force them to make the time. This shifts their attitude. Just by looking at the MAP schedule from a different perspective gives them what they need to adjust their lives in order to accommodate a session. There wouldn't be a question about working to accommodate an important meeting or class. They could do it. The mind game allows them to transfer that ability and apply it to MAP. If you're overwhelmed by this schedule thing, you might try this trick.

Of course, no amount of mind games will get you to actually schedule MAP if you really don't wish to do this kind of work. If you find you are becoming surprisingly creative about ways you can prevent yourself from having sessions, take the hint. You probably don't want to do this now. Put the book aside. At some point you'll pick it up, read it again, and find that, much to your surprise, you have no trouble scheduling those MAP sessions.

You Can't Decide If You Want to Work with MAP

When you are deciding if you would like to participate in the program, I suggest that you make a five-month commitment to MAP—and then decide after the

51

five months if you want to *continue* participating in the program. There are many things I can say about MAP and my experiences with it. But, to be honest, I can't adequately express to you in words how different and phenomenal this program is. You have to experience it for yourself. And, to appreciate what the program can do for you, you have to experience it for more than one or two sessions. After five months, you will have gone through all of the beginning schedule and established yourself in the once-a-month rhythm. I feel at that point you will be able to make a good decision. And, by that time, you will see that you really can integrate MAP into your life without causing a major upheaval to your schedule.

Chapter 4

How to Work with MAP and What Happens in a Session

I have worked with MAP personally and as part of the research and development at Perelandra since the summer of 1984. And I have gone through many different schedules with my team ranging from daily sessions to once a week or every three days. I have always allowed them to set a suggested pace, feeling that I would receive more from MAP both personally and as a researcher if I listened to my team. The scheduling for personal sessions did not correspond with specific physical or emotional "rough periods" when one might expect an increased need for MAP. Instead, they suggested an increase in sessions when my life became generally intense and it was imperative that my balance be maintained throughout.

What I would like to relate to you now are not only some of my experiences, but also suggestions based on my experiences and my work around MAP.

Here's my first suggestion: Read this chapter *frequently*

as you develop your working relationship with MAP. It has a lot of helpful information in it—too much for you to absorb in one reading. People have asked me a lot of questions about MAP over the years, and I find that ninety percent of those questions were already answered in this chapter. With this revised edition, there is even more information. So, consider this chapter your on-going support and good friend.

The sessions are always different. I can never count on a session to be one way or another, even after all this time. When *I* think something is happening in my life that warrants a difficult session, I may get a gentle, easy one. I often have tough sessions when I least expect them. If I enter a session with a complaint about my right shoulder being stiff, I may feel them working on my left foot throughout the session. After the session, my right shoulder feels fine.

Sometimes, during the easy sessions I feel absolutely nothing. I know I am connected with my team and we may be "chatting" back and forth, but I can't feel them working on me. (I have accused them of gold-bricking!) At other times, I will feel my body gently move. I even feel that I'm being turned over or that I'm floating. Of course, when I look at myself, I'm still on the bed. But had I not opened my eyes, I would never have guessed that I had not physically moved. Sometimes I feel "electrical currents" flowing throughout my body or through part of my body. Sometimes I feel tingling sensations. All these things are quite pleasant.

54

During the tough sessions, I feel pain. Sometimes—but not often—it's difficult pain. Usually the pain centers around emotional releases, and I have learned that emotional pain is truly as physically tangible as physical pain. When the pain comes, I tell my team. Then I ask if I should test for essences. Sometimes they say yes, sometimes they say it's not necessary. (If you can't "hear," this is where kinesiology testing comes in handy.) As intense as the pain may get, my team has *always* brought me full circle by the end of the session and the pain is no longer present. I have never left a session still having the pain. One of my suggestions to you, one I practice constantly, is to tell your team when pain occurs, how intense it is, and where it is located. I also tell them when the intensity either increases or decreases.

I have sometimes had a fun reaction when I was dealing with emotions in a session—the sensation that little "champagne bubbles" of energy float up through my chest and just pop out. This often makes me laugh.

Sometimes I'll be "bopping along" in my session, and all of a sudden, I'll start deep breathing spontaneously and that will go on for some minutes. And then just as suddenly, I'll stop breathing deeply. During these times, I will relax and go with the impulses.

At other times, I cry. The odd thing is that it seems as if my team has hit a "cry button," and I just start crying. Sometimes I feel the specifics of the emotion, sometimes not. Sometimes insights surface, sometimes not. I also have had insights after the session when I was just going about my day again. Something comes to mind out of the blue, and everything from the session falls into place.

Most of the time after a session, I feel fine. I have never been "left hanging" by my team. They seem to work in a rhythm that completes itself within the context of a single session. Sometimes I feel tired after a session, but a nap or a night's sleep takes care of that. Also, I usually feel vulnerable about the session itself, and I choose not to talk to anyone about the specifics. I feel very close to my team and focus our work solely with them. But I've heard from others that they like to talk about their sessions. Their problem is finding someone to talk to. It helps them integrate the sessions.

A handful of times over these past years, I have been absolutely fine after a session, and then the next day I take on a sudden, unexplainable pain that seems to come from nowhere. I have learned that at these times my body's adjustment to the work done has hit a glitch. As soon as I can, I will open a MAP session and tell them what is going on. Every time they have taken care of the problem.

Some have said that when this happens, and they only have a little time, they will quickly open a MAP coning and tell their team what is going on and that they can only give the team fifteen minutes. The team works fifteen minutes to take care of the problem. At the end of the session, the person checks for needed essences. Then, within the next twenty-four hours, they will have a regular forty-minute session in order for the team to complete their work.

Being a part-time klutz, I am sometimes prone to an accident or two. I work extensively with flower essences, so when I have an accident I immediately check myself for essences. Actually I have bottles of my ETS (Emergency Trauma Solution) on hand and, immediately after *any* accident—minor or major—I take several doses of the ETS. (For information on the ETS and how to make it, see Chapter 6.) Then I open a MAP session and tell them what I have done to myself—this time. They have neutralized wasp stings, completely eliminated a black eye (I had hit my eye on a hook and it was well on its way to being a nasty black eye in about ten minutes), and worked me through a severely sprained ankle to the point that I was walking without a limp or pain in two days. They are also whiz-bangs at getting rid of sinus headaches.

I don't ask them a lot of questions about what they are doing. I know there are some people who are using MAP and just need to know *everything*. Oftentimes these people are not yet capable of communicating directly with their team and become frustrated about not knowing exactly what is going on. Quite frankly, I don't want to know all the nuts and bolts about what my team is doing. I sense that they are working in ways that I, at best, would barely understand. Instead, I focus on how I am reacting and responding to their work—and on the results of MAP. This way, I learn more about myself, recognize what I am experiencing from MAP, and am more capable of giving my team the quality feedback they need about how I am functioning. In short, I let my MAP team do their job and I do mine.

When I first talked about MAP at a workshop, I cautioned people not to open a session if they are tired and likely to fall asleep. I still say this, but based on the letters I got back, I need to modify it a little. It is important that, whenever possible, you not come into a session in such an exhausted state that you conk out in the first five minutes. However, just about everyone who was working with MAP reported that they often fell asleep in the sessions no matter what they did. I asked Lorpuris about this, and he said that the team will put you in a sleep state at certain times when it is important for the work being done. Usually, an especially mentally active person who is getting "in the way" of the work will be put in a sleep state. When they need you to be alert, they will wake you up again. So, *your* responsibility will be to enter the MAP session when you can maintain alertness and can interact with your team. However, if you find you are going to sleep anyway, just relax about it. You have done your part by intending to be awake as you move through the session.

Sometimes you may feel you've just been fired out of a cannon! I think we have a wake-up button right next to that sleep button. The teams seem to use them both rather frequently. If you wake up with a jolt that frightens you or feels unpleasant, just tell your team and let them know you'd like something a little more gentle.

By the way, the forty-minute time for a session begins

after the coning has been opened and you have checked yourself for flower essences.

If there are other people in your family who decide to work with MAP, your session schedules will not conflict with one another. You can all have your MAP sessions at the same time. MAP isn't a doctor's office where everyone has to wait his turn. However, if more than one MAP session is going on in the house simultaneously, make sure you are not in the same room. Each person needs to be in his own room.

Sometimes people wake up during the night and feel they need a session. You can have a session in bed next to your spouse or partner *if* you can get at least a three-foot clear space between you. Your team will have difficulty with the impact of another energy field from this person if he or she—or the dog—is too close. If you don't have enough clear space, you'll have to go into another room for the session.

If the flu or any such illness is running through the family and you don't yet have it, nor do you want it, have frequent MAP sessions throughout the siege. Your team will help you maintain your balance and keep up your strength.

Don't forget that MAP can work with more than physical issues. It is important for you to also bring up any emotional stress, mental pressures, and spiritual conflicts. The PEMS levels are interrelated, and oftentimes your key to any one level hinges on your acknowledging and talking about the pains, pressures, and conflicts going on at the other three levels.

IMPORTANT: I have not needed surgery or broken any bones; consequently, I have not worked with MAP in these situations. But I have discussed this with Lorpuris, and I strongly suggest that you let common sense prevail and have needed surgery or broken bones set— and let MAP assist you during an emergency (see Chapter 6), surgery, and recovery. In short, utilize the best medical practices possible for exceptional needs requiring quick physical attention. At the same time, look to MAP for assistance in any preparation you might require and the more complex areas of repair and healing resulting from the injury or surgery.

HOW TO WORK BETTER
WITH YOUR MAP TEAM

Talking to Your Team

There are four points to remember when talking to your team.

1. Clearly define how you are feeling and your current symptoms. And don't just focus on your physical glitches. Think about any emotional stress, mental strain, or spiritual conflict. An imbalance can show up on more than one level, and it is important to work with as much of the full problem as possible. Put all symptoms "on the table."

2. Talk to your team as if they know nothing about

what is happening to you. Include everything that comes to mind as you are describing things to them.

3. Give good follow-up. After a MAP session, be aware of any changes (good ones as well as the difficult ones) that happen to you on any level, even if the change doesn't seem to have any relationship to the things you talked about in the session. When you have your next session, tell your team about these changes. They will decide if the changes had anything to do with the work and what the changes mean in relationship to that work. The important thing for you is that you recognize that there have been changes.

HINT: Unless you have an exceptional memory, I suggest that you not rely on remembering all the changes you notice after a session. Keeping a list of the changes and referring to it during the next session can make life a lot easier for you.

4. When you have no pressing symptoms and you are thinking about what to talk about in a MAP session, pick the issue that most stands out in your mind to talk about. Don't dump.

AVOID OVERLOADING A SESSION: I have written that whatever symptoms you have, tell your team. I'm not changing this. Whatever symptoms you feel before going into and during a session indicate the things you are ready to work with. However, believe it or not, there will be times when you will feel symptom-free. And you will have specific issues in mind that you would like to work on with MAP. Don't treat these issues like symptoms and throw every issue you can think of "on the table" in one session. You are going to overwhelm yourself.

Here's what you can do instead. List all the issues you'd like to work on with your team. Then, choose the most important issue to work on first, and gradually work your way down the list in future sessions. Better yet, ask your team which issue *they* recommend and get an intuitive hit or kinesiology test (if you can't hear their answer) to discern which issue should be worked on first. Once you have moved through this issue satisfactorily, review your list of issues and find out what you are to work on next. Continue doing this until there is nothing left on the list. (No need to feel you have to rush through your symptoms list. It'll keep you busy for years.)

If you overload a session by introducing too many issues, that can overload *you* as you try to comprehend all of the team's input. If you throw your team fifty balls, they may throw fifty balls back to you. The question is whether or not you are capable of catching that many all at once.

You will be constantly improving and developing your ability to communicate with your team. A major key in working with MAP well is not what your team could say to you; it is what you say to your team. What you say indicates the speed and scope of change you wish to accomplish with your team. If you can't say it, they won't work on it. They assume that if you can't say it, it is not time to work on it.

A suggestion from my experience: I've been communicating with my team since 1984. We meet often. It's not that I am in such bad shape—actually, I'm in terrific condition—but we meet to work out MAP-related issues, etc. One thing I've learned is that giving full and accurate input is an art form. It's like looking through a telescope that is constantly expanding to reveal more of the picture. When we focus on what we're seeing, we think we're seeing the whole picture. But the next time we look through the telescope, we discover there are entire areas—huge areas glaring out at us—that we were not aware of.

During one session, I asked my team to help me learn to observe my situation better and to give them better, quality input. They said to concentrate my efforts on improving the quality of my input to them—keep fine-tuning what I communicate. Over the following months, with the help of my team, I made dramatic changes in my ability to perceive a situation. Now, what I say to them is more comprehensive. For example, when I talk about something that is physically distressing, I am better able to pick up more of the nuances surrounding the distress. And I remember to add those subtle things on the other three levels that at one time I thought could never in a million years be related to the physical problem—but were. As a result, the MAP team is able to work with me in deeper, more effective ways. My movement with them has improved manyfold.

This input business is such a detailed, comprehensive art form that I don't see myself mastering it for many years to come. It is a fascinating internal journey that develops personal discipline and life tools in ways that are simply unimaginable. I recommend it to all of you. Just ask your team to help you improve your perception and ability to communicate what you see, think, and feel. Then, focus on giving your team the best input you can give. You'll see the changes. And have patience with yourself. Give yourself time to learn.

INCLUDE THE POSITIVE: Surprise your MAP team. Tell them the good stuff that's going on in your life—and include any good insights you have had. By concentrating on the tough stuff, we are implying that only the tough stuff in our lives molds and moves us. This is nuts! So give the good stuff a hearing. (Does this sound like I'm standing on the sidelines madly cheering you on?!)

FEELING STUCK: You've brought up a problem that you and your team have been working on. You feel like you've done everything but the problem remains. You feel like you've hit a wall and don't know what else to say or do. Well, you *have* hit a wall, but it's not with your team. It's a wall inside yourself. Ask your team to give you insight about what to do. The insight will help you move through or around the wall and you'll be on track again.

Better yet, do a MAP/Calibration around the fact that you have hit a wall either with your work with MAP in

general or with a specific issue. (See Chapter 5 on MAP/Calibration.)

A NOTE ABOUT HEARING YOUR TEAM: I suggest that you relax about this. *Many* people don't get any kind of communication in a session. You don't need to hear or feel anything to participate in MAP. Your verification that something is really happening will be in the changes you feel around issues you've brought up in the sessions. Your whole focus will be on how you are responding.

I know everyone would prefer to hear and see their teams. But whether one does depends on the range of function of the sensory system. It's as simple as that. Desire, deep concentration, worry, and wishes won't make a difference. As I said, hearing and seeing the teams depends on our range of sensory function. When I am in a MAP session, I can hear my team clearly, but I can't see them. From talking about this issue in the workshops, I find out that a handful of people in the class can both hear and see. A larger number can experience one or the other, but not both. Equal in number to this second group are those who can neither hear, see, nor sense their team. These people are always surprised to learn how many are in the same boat as they are. Many of these people say they feel their team communicates with them by giving them intuitive insights as they go about their normal daily schedule.

What has been made clear is that most people who start out sensing nothing gradually expand their sensory

systems to where, six months to a year down the road, they can indeed hear and/or see their teams.

Kinesiology is the bridge to your team if you can't hear them. As long as you know how to use kinesiology, you will be able to get answers to any of the questions you might have about your health and health practices. All you need to do is formulate the questions in a simple yes/no format.

NOTE: Communication with your team will be more accurate and have greater range if you use kinesiology instead of relying on intuition. It's tough to get clear, precise, and complex information through intuition unless you are well-disciplined in this area.

IMPORTANT: Many people who have had trouble feeling a clear yes/no response with their kinesiology asked their teams to help them achieve the needed (and desired) clarity. They report that the kinesiology problems cleared up quickly and easily. So, let your team help you with your fears and difficulties as you develop this tool.

The MAP Coning and Team

ABOUT THE MAP CONING: A MAP coning is very precise, and it is set up as the MAP Unit and nature wish. It is their program. (For more information about conings, see Appendix A.) It has been set up to give anyone who wishes quality health care in a perfectly safe environment. It was researched and developed for seven years prior to our offering the program to the

public. Please consider this if you are toying with the idea of changing the makeup of the coning or how the program is set up. Some people have consciously worked in interlevel ways with souls prior to MAP. They feel that they must include these souls in the MAP coning. This is not true and it is also not helpful. MAP is a specialized coning designed and set up for comprehensive health care for those of us on the Earth level. It's not helpful to "load" others into the MAP coning who are not participating in the program. Anyone who should be a part of your medical team will automatically be included when the team is formed during the scanning session. If you would like to know if a soul you have already known and worked with is also part of your MAP team, just ask your team.

If, despite all that I've said, you feel compelled to alter the MAP coning or change any part of the program, always consult your team first—as a matter of courtesy, if for no other reasons. Get their okay. And know that any approved changes in your coning or program are made just for you and are not to be passed on to others.

If you arbitrarily decide that you would like to set up the coning with different members or refer to the MAP-coning members by names that really do not apply to them, you will not have a MAP coning. Instead, you will have a coning comprised of those you have called in. And whatever happens while you have this coning activated will not be a MAP session. I am not saying that bad things will happen to you. I am only saying that when you arbitrarily change the composition of this coning, you no longer have a MAP coning. You may have a peaceful, even interesting session, but it will not be a MAP session. (For how to set up other conings, see Appendix A.)

Also, some people feel more comfortable if they include Jesus Christ in their MAP coning. Jesus Christ is a member of the White Brotherhood and will be glad to join your coning. But He is not part of the medical teams and will not be working with you medically. He will be present in a supportive capacity.

Half of the MAP team originates from the White Brotherhood. (The other half is nature.) "Brotherhood," in this instance, means "all"—as in "all life." It does not mean "men." Do not assume your team is made up solely of men. But, if you feel you do have a bunch of men—or a bunch of women!—and this makes you uncomfortable, say something to your team. Their feelings won't be hurt. They will adjust the energy and the makeup of your team appropriately.

Also, the MAP teams operate beyond time and space. There is no issue, as far as they are concerned, about your needing a session at 3 A.M. You are not waking them up and you are not pestering them. Have sessions at a time that is convenient to you.

In this same area, your team doesn't wake you up for a session. You will not be disturbed by them. They may not exist in time and space, but they are well aware of those dynamics—and that *we* exist in time and space.

ABOUT YOUR HIGHER SELF: When I instruct you to connect with and disconnect from your higher self, I do not mean to imply that you haven't been connected all along. You cannot exist without a strong, functioning bond with your higher self! However, for MAP and other coning work, you temporarily expand the range of connection so that you can have *clear, conscious interaction* between your higher self and your conscious self. It takes a lot of physical energy to maintain this expanded connection. For your balance and well-being, it is important to readjust the connection back to your normal range once you have completed the work that required the special connection in the first place. If you don't do this (or you forget), you will experience an energy drain.

Some people have ignored my warnings about this. They want to be connected to their higher selves in this expanded range all the time. However, if they had been physically capable of maintaining such a connection indefinitely, they would not have had to expand the range in the first place. They would be automatically functioning in the more expanded range. It only takes a day or two to feel the effects of trying to maintain this connection. They feel run down, exhausted, and sometimes lethargic. If you should ignore my warnings and find yourself in the same situation (and you wish to get out of it), just disconnect from your higher self in the usual way. This will immediately adjust the connection to your normal day-to-day range. Then get some rest and eat a couple of high-protein meals. In a day or two you will be back to your old self—and glad for it!

Problem Sessions

SEEKING INSTANT PERFECTION: Some people who are doing MAP have told me that they gave everything over to their teams. Basically they made a blanket statement at some point in their MAP development (usually right at the beginning) that the team was to do whatever was needed to make them "perfect." But then they were disappointed because not a whole lot was happening.

MAP doesn't accept that kind of blanket surrendering. You are creating a partnership with them and not surrendering yourself as a child to a parent. Plus, when *we* say "take it all and do everything" we don't necessarily realize what this implies. MAP requires that you consciously and knowingly request their assistance in specific areas. If there are areas in need of assistance that you don't understand or know about, the team will gently help bring these areas into your consciousness so that you can make appropriate decisions. How you proceed tells your team in what directions you'd like to go. Try to remember that your MAP team is extraordinarily expansive in what it knows and can do. Therefore, you must indicate to them *your* directions and pace so that they work with you specifically within the framework that *you* define.

APPROPRIATE SESSION ENVIRONMENTS: Most of you wouldn't arrange for a surgeon to do a biopsy on you while you are in your car driving to work. (Notice I hedged my bets and said "most.") You and the surgeon would prefer the work be done in an appropriate environment. The same is true with your MAP team. They don't want to work on you while you are driving to work. (By the way, I'm using this driving example because someone boasted to me that they actually did this.) Your MAP team doesn't ask for a lot. But they do insist that you be alone, alert for the session, and unoccupied with anything else during the session. If you open a session while in an inappropriate setting, the team will not work on you. They'll just wait quietly until you close the coning.

MAP IS A MEDICAL PROGRAM: These teams will not make real estate or employment recommendations, they will not focus on how your business is doing, they will not assist you in your campaign for public office, and they don't care about what your local city council is deciding. It is a *medical* program, and it deals only with medical issues. If you like working with a coning, and you would like to set one up for a nonmedical area in your life, please do so. (See Appendix A.) But don't bring it to MAP.

MAP IS A MEDICAL PROGRAM FOR HUMANS—NOT ANIMALS: The team members are not veterinarians. They specialize in the human body. If you wish to assist an animal in a similar program, use the Nature Healing Coning for Animals. (See Chapter 11.) This was designed specifically for animals and is as effective for them as MAP is for us.

ANIMALS IN YOUR SESSIONS: Animals absorb stressful

human energy patterns. If you've ever had an argument with someone while your dog or cat was in the same room, and then watched the animal's behavior change right before your eyes, you know what I'm talking about. A lot of deep work goes on with you during a MAP session. Just because an animal wants to be near you while you are quietly sitting or lying down does not mean that animal wants or needs to experience your MAP session. And your team doesn't want to work with you while you have a cat plunked on your chest or lap. The two energy fields are going to commingle, and this isn't helpful for your team. Do you, your team, and your animals a favor and don't include animals in your sessions.

MAP JUNKIES: MAP is fantastic. There's no doubt about this. Most people who experience MAP say they have never experienced anything like it in their lives. But some people have gotten hooked on the program and have jumped off the deep end with it. They have sessions two, three, or four times a day. And they insist that the sessions remain open for hours at a time.

MAP is a program that was designed to be integrated in a *balanced* manner into your life. It is not designed for taking over your life. The teams deal with a MAP junkie with terrific patience. They will work in a focused manner to help that person achieve a sense of appropriate balance in his life. At some point, the person will be hit with common sense and, hopefully, work with their team in a more balanced way. I say "hopefully" because sometimes the person will overreact and reject MAP altogether. They blame their "addiction" on MAP.

If you do not have a compelling reason to have daily sessions, and you feel you might be a junkie and wish to achieve a more balanced relationship with MAP, just talk to your team about this. Describe your feelings about the program, how you feel when you are in a session, and how you feel when you are not in a session. Let them work with you consciously on this issue.

Comprehending What's Happening

You don't have to be able to hear your team talk to receive understanding about what is going on with you. MAP comprehension comes from insights and understanding that happen in various ways. Don't assume your team is going to write things down for you on golden tablets. The insights usually occur within the context of your everyday life. Often, you may be walking along a week or so after a session, thinking about absolutely nothing or humming some song when, all of a sudden, out of nowhere, you'll have an insight. It doesn't hit you hard. But suddenly a light goes on. It's a quiet thing. Also, pay close attention to your dreams. You may get a lot of insight and understanding this way, as well.

Comprehension often relies on new thinking. You may not be able to comprehend what's new with your old thinking. If you are working on a health issue (physical, emotional, mental, or spiritual) with MAP, this implies

73

that you are having difficulty with that issue—otherwise, you wouldn't bother bringing it up. The resolution of many issues requires new thinking, new insights. The MAP team will "slip" these to you in unexpected ways. This catches you off guard so you won't mentally reject the insight or alter it and then fit it comfortably into your old thinking.

Don't be afraid to tell your team that you are totally at a loss about something. Actually, I say this to my team pretty often. It tends to be just the thing I need to admit that will then break up the logjam. I find that it's as good for us to articulate how much we don't know as it is how much we do know.

Also, don't assume you have to understand everything. You only have to understand what's relevant. Some things can occur in a session that are part of the issue being worked on but are not key to it. In order to understand the issue, you do not need to understand this one thing. Trust that your team will make sure you get the insight and information that is relevant to the issue—and let the rest float on by you.

A REMINDER ABOUT REPORTING YOUR INSIGHTS: Once you have an insight, be sure you report it to your team in the next session. This way, your team knows you "got it," and while listening to you, they can tell how much of the insight you were able to grasp. This is how you communicate the pace and scope of your movement through issues. So, be clear and concise with your descriptions and understandings. (This is another reason why it's important to stay awake, if you can, during a MAP session. You really need to talk.)

Also, I pay attention to whatever pops into my head as I describe an insight to my team and include this in what I'm saying. Sometimes an event that occurred in my past will pop up and, as I describe it, certain emotions surface. The old event and the insight may not be related at all. But the emotions the old event activated may be crucial to understanding the insight.

Reaction to Sessions

You had a MAP session, came out of it fine, and took flower essences. Then, sometime within the next twenty four to thirty-six hours you began to feel unwell. You sense you are having a "reaction" to something that occurred during the session. You are scheduled to have another session next week. Here's what to do. Open a session as soon as possible and let them know exactly how you feel. When this happens to me, I usually feel like "something slipped" and I need to have the team "put it back into position." After this session, you'll be back on track. Before closing the session, ask if your schedule has changed. Don't assume they still want to see you in a week.

IF YOU HAVE NO TIME FOR A SESSION: Have a quick session. Let's say you have fifteen minutes before you have to leave the house. (Or a fifteen-minute break at work, and you can have privacy during this time.

Bathrooms are good for this.) Open a session and let them know exactly how you feel and that you only have fifteen minutes (or however long you have). Have the session and check for essences, if you have them available. *When you do a quick session, you must follow it up with a regular forty-minute session within twenty-four hours.* After the follow-up regular session, ask if your schedule from your original session (the one before the quick session) has changed.

The following is from an article published in our newsletter, *Perelandra Voices.*

I began doing MAP during Christmas vacation. It was difficult to return to work and put my energy in outer things. These sessions are, in some ways, hard work. My first day back at work, I got home beaten and frazzled after a long day. I was so exhausted—mentally, physically, emotionally—that I was unable to cope and in a state of panic and totally overwhelmed. I didn't have time to do a full MAP session. My husband was due home in 20 minutes. So I called a quick MAP session of 20 minutes (I didn't know if this was "legal," but I had to do something.) The first five minutes I sobbed hard, then felt sedated again. About halfway through, I felt a sudden intense electrical shock go through a joint of my ring finger—it jerked my arm off the bed and made me cry out. Then, nothing else. At the end of 20 minutes, I was in a totally different state. I was still a little tired, but I did all the things I needed to do that evening without strain, anxiety, or fatigue. On the contrary, I felt emotionally calm and peaceful. This may not sound like much to you, but it is a true miracle to me.

E. R., Oregon

Tough Sessions

To write about this effectively, I must lean on my personal background and my resulting experiences in this area.

When I was twelve years old, I became what is known today as a throwaway child. (If you would like details about this, see *Behaving As If the God In All Life Mattered*.) This led to a number of years of difficult experiences. I'm being a little glib here because the details are not the issue right now. Suffice it to say that those early years, prior to being sent out on my own and after, were most unpleasant.

Part of my coming to terms with this time and these experiences was to process what happened, how I felt about it then and how I feel about it as an adult. As a result of this reflection, I reached a level of internal balance. I was happy and certainly quite functional. I did not feel as if those early years weighed me down at all.

Another way to look at the internal balance that I felt is to say that as I addressed and moved through each issue, a scaffolding was created inside me. Each issue became part of the scaffold. When I could feel internal balance, the scaffold was fully formed and served to give me a new supportive strength. I had taken what at one time was destructive to me, worked it over, turned it around, and created from these same experiences a scaffold of strength. I don't believe that this scaffold phenomenon is unique to me. On the contrary, I feel that

77

this happens inside each of us as we address certain painful life issues. We can choose for our life experiences to create a scaffold of weakness and destructiveness, or we can take those same experiences, turn them around and create a strong, supportive scaffold with them.

For many years, my scaffold gave me a good, strong, workable balance. Then in 1982, I expanded my life in a way that required that I seek a new level of balance. One result of this is MAP. The heretofore perfectly fine scaffold had to be shifted to accommodate the new balance. That meant that it had to be dismantled. Each piece had to be either modified and placed differently, or released altogether. And sometimes, this can be tough.

This scaffold work is a real, physical dynamic. It is not some mental construct I've invented. We must physically, emotionally, mentally, and spiritually shift in order to modify and reposition or release these scaffold pieces. From this, we create a new scaffold that strengthens and supports us on our new level in life.

MAP creates a safe environment for you. And every cell in your body knows this. So, where you might normally resist making these deep and challenging changes without MAP, you will most likely be inclined to actually say yes to them because of MAP. This program gives you a feeling of both support and safety. And there couldn't be a more appropriate environment for you to face these changes head on and make them.

An important point about scaffold sessions: You will not enter into this kind of tough session unless you are both ready and willing. Your team does not drag you kicking and screaming into a tough session. You may not consciously know what is ahead of you, but you have consciously put yourself in position for this, and your heart and soul have said yes. The teams do not trick you into a tough session. All they do is support you in every way as *you* prepare for and move through these sessions.

You might have some intense reactions in scaffold sessions when these pieces are being addressed, modified, repositioned, or released. You can experience intense physical pain, either generally throughout your body or localized in an area that is related to the scaffold piece being worked on. You may have a sudden and deep feeling of anguish descend on you, and you don't know what's causing it. You may feel the need to scream. Or the need to vomit. (My personal favorite.) You may feel unable to move or speak. And often, you will feel a strong desire to curl up in a fetal position. (It's important that you do not actually curl up. Remain in your usual session position.)

I have never known beforehand when I am going to have a tough session. They just happen. When they have occurred, my team kept me in the session for ninety minutes. This allowed them the time to make sure the changes were complete and stabilized. I have never come out of a session feeling that I was left hanging. Each time I have had a tough session, I have come out of the session feeling a deep sense of peace.

In my ten years working with MAP, I'd say I've had a total of fifteen sessions I would call tough. Most of them

79

occurred in the early years. I haven't had any in a number of years. But I don't rule out the possibility of having tough sessions in the future. I have no fears about them. I know I'm perfectly safe.

Another thing: Most of the time I cannot identify what specific piece of my scaffold is being worked on. I can be having all kinds of reactions, but they're not connected with any piece of information that would give me insight as to what is occurring. I also don't ask for insight. If it's important for me, my team will make sure I get it. If it's not important—and most of the time it's not—I don't want to be bothered. As far as I am concerned, I'm ready to make the shift and I just want to get on with that process.

By the way, not all scaffold sessions are tough. Some of the pieces move into place effortlessly. As I said, tough sessions don't occur often. But when they do, they can be quite something.

What to do if you should find yourself in a tough session: First of all, automatically assume you need to extend the session to last ninety minutes rather than forty minutes. Second, don't panic. You are in the best hands and you are fine. Tell the team everything you are feeling—every physical, emotional, mental, and spiritual pain. Tell them when you want to curl up, when you feel so mentally restless you could scream, when you feel chilled or overheated. I also include when I'd like to punch out my team for this session I'm in. It gives them something to think about, and I feel better for having made the threat! All of this gives them feedback about how you are doing and where they need to shore you up. If you have to vomit or go to the bathroom, tell your team. They'll put everything on hold while you take care of business. The ninety minutes does not include a bathroom break, so you will need to add this to your session time.

After one of these sessions, you might want a nap and you might feel vulnerable. You will also feel peaceful. Later, if you have any discomfort resulting from the session, see your team as soon as possible. Flower essences support this process well, so make sure you test for them.

Frightening Experiences

The MAP teams do not do things to scare you half to death. I've heard many refer to their teams as "gentle" and "loving" beyond belief. MAP teams do not throw things around the room or at you. They do not steal money from your wallet, or keep your body in perpetual sessions and refuse to "let go" even though you beg them to. They do not take over your life or tell you what to do or say. They do not wake you up every morning at some ungodly hour. In fact, they don't wake you up at all. Nor do they rip flowers out of your garden. These are all actual accusations people have made against their MAP teams. Here's some more of what they don't do: They don't automatically connect with you without permission, solve business problems, discourse on local government issues, heal animals, work on others without the other person's *conscious* permission, and they won't suggest that for the betterment of your soul you should become a tree.

This is not an intergalactic street gang you've teamed up with. They have the highest integrity. They will not work with you in harmful ways—and they will not harm you, period.

Now, if you have frightening experiences, MAP is not doing them to you. You are doing them to yourself. You are scared beyond words, and being in MAP isn't helping the situation. If you are having this experience, tell MAP immediately. If your fears and frightening experiences have not disappeared within one or two more sessions, *stop doing MAP altogether*—and right away. You are fighting yourself and you are not capable, in your present condition, of clearly discerning what is going on in a session. You are translating it in terrible, frightening ways. You need to do more personal balancing work around the causes of your fears to be able to perceive a session accurately before re-entering MAP.

People who have serious victimization, paranoid, or schizophrenic tendencies are especially vulnerable. Although MAP is perfectly capable of assisting people with these problems, the MAP program itself can exacerbate their problems. In these instances, MAP is not for them. Good, qualified counseling or therapy plus flower essences is the way to go in these situations.

Another issue involves constantly hearing voices. MAP teams usually work quietly, unless you ask them

something or are talking to them. They are not chatter-
boxes by any means. A couple of people have said that
their teams talk all the time to them—within a session
and outside a session. They say they have asked the
teams to stop, but they won't. And then these people tell
me that their teams are telling them to do odd things.
One fellow was "told" to have an affair with his neigh-
bor. Another was being "told" to fuse with and become
one with the aforementioned tree, and once they did
this, they would be able to serve the world in new and
wondrous ways.

I hate to disappoint you folks out there, but MAP
teams are actually quite reasonable in both what they
talk about and how they say it. They really don't sound
like a bunch of New Age freakouts. Their demeanor is
polite, kind, caring, respectful, supportive—and always
professional.

What's happening with these people is that they are
hearing themselves. MAP has gotten them both excited
and scared, and they've fallen off into fantasy conversations that they attribute to MAP because the talks sound
just like what they imagine a MAP team would say. And
they think the teams are "saying" exactly what the person wants to hear.

Sometimes, these people are so unhappy with their
lives and yearn to do something "significant." The
yearning becomes so great that it trips them over the
edge, and they begin to hear voices telling them how
great they are and what they need to do to help save the
world. Again, they are hearing themselves.

Here's what to do in this situation: Tell your team you're being hounded by voices. Also tell your team you plan not to take the voices seriously anymore. (And then don't take them seriously anymore! Don't do anything or say anything based on what these voices are saying. In short, render them powerless.) From that point on, your team will work with you without saying a word. They will also not communicate with you through kinesiology. Most likely, if you have been using kinesiology, you are not sure if you are controlling the testing. By the team maintaining silence in these two areas, you won't have the problem of trying to discern who is talking. If they need to get something across to you, they will do it in another way, but it won't be verbal. Then they will work with you to move you into a more balanced position where you will no longer hear voices.

You won't be able to ask them about a session schedule because they are no longer talking to you. So, plan to have weekly sessions until the voices disappear. Then have sessions twice a month for the next two months. After this, have sessions monthly.

IMPORTANT: There is a difference between a tough scaffold session and a frightening experience. A scaffold session can be tough because of a strong reaction or response you are having as a result of the work being done. A frightening experience usually involves some perceived attack either by the team or some outside force. Because of the coning, no force outside the coning can disturb you in anyway. You are fully protected.

Trying to Control Your Team

Some people try to control or "corner" their MAP team. These people want something or need to make sure they are right about something. They usually attempt to control their team by how they ask the team questions. For example, if a person really wants to have MAP sessions three times a day, he will ask questions about his schedule that will ensure that the answer leaves open the possibility of super-frequent sessions. For example, rather than asking how often he should have sessions, he will ask if having sessions as often as he would like is okay. If he is discerning the answer through kinesiology, the answer will most likely be positive. It's okay. What the team is really saying is that it is okay, but it is not needed nor is it particularly useful. By the way the question is phrased, the person hasn't allowed for this kind of input from the team. In order to get full information, you may have to ask a series of questions. You ask the main question, then ask additional questions that allow for any modification or qualification of the main question. The way to continue the schedule questioning with your team would be to also ask if frequent sessions are *needed*. Now you've given your team a chance to say "okay, but not needed."

The team will not work on you in useless or harmful ways. The people who ask these kinds of limiting or controlling questions can open a MAP session as often as they like. But, most likely, the most significant issue the team will be working on is your addiction to MAP sessions.

When asking for information from your team, look at how you are phrasing the questions and see if you are presenting them in a manner that supports your own desires. In short, are you being honest in what you are asking. In this kind of situation, you are not controlling your team, you are controlling yourself. Your team knows exactly what you are trying to do. And, as I said, they will work with you to overcome this situation, but they will not participate in your efforts to control them.

Another issue occurs when you wish to control the answer by asking your team a question and then supplying only the options or actions you desire to follow. For example, you have verified that your team is suggesting a change in diet. You can't hear them tell you the changes, so the only way to get the information is by using kinesiology. You test a list of things that are in your current diet. You are asking the question, "Do I eliminate this item?" That's all fine, except that you chose to leave a few things off your list—like the daily three martinis and pint of Ben and Jerry's Heath Bar Crunch ice cream. In this situation, MAP will answer you according to the best of the options you have given. However, it may not be the best option overall for you. When you give options, remember to add at the end of your list "none of the above." This allows your team to get across to you that you are going to have to expand your options if you want the best answer.

Keep questions short, clear, clean, and honest. If you

are using kinesiology, you will need to ask them in a simple yes/no format. The simplicity of this format is helpful in maintaining clarity whether we are using kinesiology or hearing our team directly—and simplicity makes it easier to spot our creative attempts at control.

Session Aerobics and Sleep

SESSION AEROBICS: I've written about not moving physically or crossing your limbs during the session. Let me qualify this. It's important that you remain physically quiet during a session. Don't toss and turn. Don't cross your arms over your chest, and don't cross your legs. But sometimes you'll sense a specific movement— like a clear impulse to move in a specific manner. This probably is something your team wants you to do and may be related to an adjustment they are working on. Go with the motion. If you can hear your team, ask them if they'd like you to do the movement. If you are communicating through the use of kinesiology, ask the same question and test for the answer. If you do neither, but have a strong sense of a well-defined movement, go with your gut instinct, tell your team what you are about to do—and do it. These movements are not complicated. Nor do they last long. It's not as if you are going to do tough calisthenics for forty minutes. (And it doesn't include jumping up and running to the store for a six-pack!)

SLEEP: I'm repeating this in several places because it is

such an issue with people. Go into the session wide awake. If you fall asleep during the session, don't worry about it. You have fulfilled your responsibility entering it awake, alert, and capable of remaining that way. But if you do fall asleep, despite these efforts, it is most likely a reaction to the work your team is doing. Or, your team needs to "get you out of the way" mentally while they work. Intelligent, inquisitive people often konk out during their sessions. Most likely, they were too active mentally and were interfering with the work that was being done. (I haven't met anyone yet who hasn't fallen asleep in a MAP session—myself included.)

If you wake up and realize that the session was probably over two hours ago, or it's the next morning and you never closed the session, it's okay. Your team won't send you a bill for time and a half. Close the coning now, and test for essences. You haven't inconvenienced your team. Remember, they operate beyond time and space, so your clock is not an issue to anyone but you.

If you tend to go to sleep and need to make sure your session doesn't run over a certain time, set an alarm clock for yourself. Just make sure you are not cutting your forty-minute session short.

Menopause and Gynecology

Menopause is a natural cycle and is therefore well understood by both nature and the White Brotherhood. It

88

need not be a time of internal chaos because it is a change that (naturally) has its own unique order and organization. But it can feel chaotic if its order and organization (balance) is off. If you read the *Co-Creative Definitions* (Appendix E), you'll see that nature supplies all of reality's order, organization, and life vitality.

As we women approach the menopause years (or *feel* we are entering that time), we can open a MAP/Calibration session and request that we be prepared for the changes so that we can enter the time in appropriate balance. (But, be prepared! This may require some lifestyle changes such as in your diet, exercise, and drinking habits!) Once requesting the help of your team, ask if you are to have a MAP/Calibration *series* of sessions specifically for menopause preparation. If so, get that schedule. It may extend over months, even longer.

As we move through menopause, we can keep in close contact with our MAP/Calibration team to maintain the unique balance that menopause requires. We can talk about all the changes as they occur, our reactions and perceptions. And we can talk about all the dumb things people say about menopause that bother us. Our teams assist us as we maintain the balance needed to experience a meaningful and healthy life change. Menopause does not have to be a chamber of horrors. (NOTE: MAP/Calibration can, in like manner, be helpful for achieving and maintaining balance during the menstrual cycle, as well.)

Also, I have asked in MAP/Calibration sessions to receive understanding about what menopause really is for us and how to better understand and view it. For me, this has sidestepped the assumptions, myths, and medical misknowledge that are associated with menopause. I must say that this experience has been deeply rewarding, and I recommend it to other women.

I also recommend this kind of MAP/Calibration to men who would like to understand more about what is really happening with their partners and how they (the men) fit into this picture.

One other related point for men: Their chemistry also changes when they are in their forties and fifties. MAP can assist men with these changes, as well.

The following is an article written for our newsletter by a woman who worked with her team on the issue of estrogen replacement therapy.

My gynecologist put me on estrogen therapy about two years ago. A competent physician, and respectful, he suggested I kinesiology test the regimen—the frequency, not the dosage. I am unhappy taking manufactured hormones. So I asked my MAP team, "Do I need to take the hormone today?" and got a positive. Now I check every day. I record when the answer is negative and when it turns positive. The hormone has a palpable effect. I always feel better, but I just hate taking medicine. My team indicated I would be on this regimen for months. So I set up a log to keep track.

Prior to involving my MAP team, my physician proposed two weeks on and two weeks off. But I became grumpy and miserable on the two weeks off. Since I teach, I didn't want to take it out on my students. So I tried it two weeks on—one week off. No luck. After day three, I was miserable. Finally, the light dawned. I asked my team; and behold, I got help. My most sincere thanks to you, your associates and the Perelandra Staff for making access to these new dimensions.

J. R., Pennsylvania

The next article from the newsletter is by a woman who worked with MAP for a gynecological problem.

I have been greatly helped by MAP. I had been spotting at mid-cycle for a year. I wasn't concerned because it was minimal and occurred only at ovulation. Then one day I had heavy bleeding and cramping in my cervix. This did make me take notice. My body was trying to tell me something that I needed to address. I immediately opened a MAP coning and was told to test for flower essences and have a MAP session. I cannot describe how comforted I felt during this entire four- to five-day process. I was assured I didn't need medical treatment. I also understood this was a healing process to release old trauma from my body.

Fifteen years ago, I had been biopsied for cervical dysplasia. As I was in the MAP session, all the emotions held in at that time came to the surface. I sobbed with the pain of feeling so alone during that ordeal. I also relived the humiliation of the procedures. I was literally almost yanked off the table during the biopsy. The tissue did not want to be taken out and yet the doctor insisted on doing that. Then there were the follow-up treatments of tissue being frozen (cryosurgery) and later cauterized. I felt awful about being disconnected from a part of my body, angry at my partner for the lack of support, frightened and humiliated by the procedures. And I had a terrible sense of loneliness. As this overwhelming loneliness arose, I asked to be comforted so I would not feel so alone this time. I truly felt I was held in loving arms. I still had to feel the pain, but there was not the isolation that had previously existed. I was told to meet the next morning for a MAP session. This continued for four consecutive days. Each day we met for a MAP session, I received the healing support of my MAP team and the flower essences. By the end of the four days, the bleeding had subsided and the sensations of pressure and cramping in my cervix had pretty much abated.

There were lessons to learn as I saw the flower essences that came up. I saw areas of my life where I was asked to take more responsibility for myself. I could see connections that had to be made for healing to occur.

I felt very much at peace during this healing process. My attention was drawn inward, and I felt able to be with my body and not be fearful about what was occurring. There actually was a feeling of sweetness about it: the amazing support and love I was receiving, the sense of coming back to my body, and of being able to nurture this very traumatized part of myself. I often had spontaneous images of a very healthy cervix come up. The support I received allowed me to feel the absolute naturalness of this unfolding process so I was able to cooperate fully and easily.

This is the first cycle I have had since this experience. I am so pleased that I did not have any breakthrough bleeding, the first time in 15 months! I can honestly say that I can feel a difference in this part of my body. The trauma has been released. My MAP team and I just celebrated the anniversary of our first year, and I feel honored and pleased to see myself entering more and more into a co-creative relationship with them. I appreciate the perceptual changes that allow me to take more responsibility for myself and contribute to healing the planet.

M. L., California

I added the following editor's note with this article:

Make sure you feel comfortable and at ease about *not* seeking regular medical help when your MAP team says it's not necessary. This is only a suggestion from your team. If you would feel more comfortable going to a regular physician, do it. If nothing else, the visit will put your mind at ease.

Just prior to the doctor's appointment, open a MAP coning. Tell your team where you are going and the physician's specialty, if he or she has one. Ask the team to monitor your visit. Then, right after the appointment or sometime later that day, have a MAP session and let your team continue the physician's work in ways that are appropriate for you.

If you don't have a MAP session immediately after returning from the doctor's office, ask your team if you should close down the MAP coning. They may wish to continue monitoring you, depending on your reaction to the visit and the state of your health. If they wish you to leave the coning open, find out how long it is to stay open. Then close the coning at the appropriate time.

If your team does not need the coning to be left open, close it down after you return home and re-open it later when you are ready to do the "post–doctor's" session.

Accidents and MAP

You've had an accident. You are still conscious, and you must go to the hospital emergency room. Open an emergency MAP session. The full process is given in Chapter 6 and the easy-reference steps are in Chapter 8. I recommend that you read Chapter 6 several times to become familiar with the process so that you can recall it in an emergency without having to dig for the book. You might even open the Emergency MAP coning several times just to practice. And make sure you have your ETS easily available for emergencies.

While you recuperate from an accident, have frequent MAP sessions. If you can't get scheduling information from your team because you can't do kinesiology testing and/or can't hear them, just have a session each day as you move through the initial recuperation stages. Also, tell them what therapy you are getting because of the accident.

EMERGENCY MAP FOR OTHERS IN NEED: The full process and information for setting up or surrogating a session for someone else who is in an emergency situation is in Chapter 6. It's easy to set the session up for someone, but there is one major, ethical issue: You must have the person's *conscious* permission to set up the session. You cannot throw a MAP team in someone else's lap. Nor can you throw someone unwittingly into MAP's lap.

If you feel you would like to offer MAP to someone in need, if the chance should arise, take time to think about how you would explain MAP to someone else who doesn't know about it or wouldn't normally be attracted to such a thing. Be careful about what words you use. Make it short, to the point and inoffensive. Try it out on others a few times and modify your explanation according to the reactions you get from these people.

IF A PERSON IS IN A COMA: It is just as crucial that you receive permission from them as it would be if they were conscious. Here's what to do: Treat the person as if he/she was conscious and fully capable of hearing you. Explain MAP. Speak audibly and softly to the person.

Then set up for surrogate kinesiology testing (see Appendix B) and ask simple yes/no questions. "Do you understand what I'm explaining?" "Would you like me to explain it again?" "Do I need to be clearer?" "Would you like me to set up a MAP coning for you?" If the answer to the last question is "no," you need to back off. If "yes," set up a surrogate Emergency MAP coning. (See Chapter 6.)

At one of the MAP workshops, a woman explained that her adult daughter had been in a coma for years due to a car accident. The mother began using MAP and felt that it was just the thing her daughter needed. She did not bother to explain MAP or get permission from her daughter to open a coning for her. The best way to describe what happened when the mother opened the session is that the daughter fought it. She didn't know what was happening to her. So she became restless and agitated in extraordinary ways. The mother remembered what I had written about this situation and talked to her daughter about MAP just as if her daughter were conscious and could hear. Immediately the daughter calmed down. She's now out of the coma and talks to her mother about the things she sees her MAP team doing for her. She can describe her team in detail, too.

The mother explained that she was talking about her experience in a public workshop because she wanted to make sure others, who have the best intentions, just as she did, pay attention to this permission business before opening a MAP coning for someone.

LONG DISTANCE MAP SESSIONS: Don't try to set up a long-distance session for someone, even if you have permission. These sessions require that the person have support from you. Like MAP for children, you need to be in the room and ready to test the person for flower essences both during and after the session. You also have to ask any pertinent questions. To set up a long distance session basically leaves the other person in the dark and unsupported. It is not an appropriate thing to do.

ABOUT ACCIDENTS AND MAP: Everyone who works at Perelandra has also "joined" MAP. We have in their files the code name for their team in case there's an accident. In a family or group situation that is MAP-friendly, you might consider recording everyone's code name to use during emergencies.

Keeping Your Team Informed

Keep your team up to date on current health issues. For example, when a flu epidemic hits your area, tell your team. They do not keep themselves up on *your* current events. You will have to supply this information.

If you are frightened about something like AIDS, or you know someone who has AIDS or has died from the disease, talk to your team about it. (And talk to your friend who has AIDS or is HIV-positive about MAP!) Even if you are not at risk, the fact that you have a fear about AIDS (or any public health issue) can compromise your PEMS (physical, emotional, mental, and spiritual) balance. And if you are in a situation where you are at risk, keep your team abreast of any feelings that you have. There is a strong link between your immune system and your state of mind.

Here is a personal example: Seven out of eight members of my immediate family died of cancer. Even though I have distanced myself from patterns that might have contributed to their cancer, and even though I have a good personal attitude and strength, I still hit an internal panic button if anything even slightly suspicious happens to me. I pay attention to those panic-button messages and I immediately inform my team. Just talking about it is helpful. But apart from this, telling my team about it is part of my responsibility to keep them well informed about what's happening to me physically *and* emotionally.

CAUTION: I strongly advise that you not ask your team emotionally charged questions like, "Do I have cancer?" Your ability to accurately perceive their answer is questionable—whether you are using kinesiology or another method for "hearing" your team. In these situations, it would be better for you and your team if you got a sound diagnosis from a medical doctor whom you trust. And, just like the allopathic doctors tell us, MAP also feels second and third opinions are valuable. Your team already knows if you have a serious problem. It doesn't need the diagnosis. However, it needs your cooperation and understanding of the situation in order to effectively work with you. Getting a diagnosis that has been verified by one or two other doctors moves you through the process of receiving a good foundation of information from which you can work with your team. It's an invaluable education process for you and will help you ask the right questions and give the right information to your team as you move through a treatment program. Also—and this is equally important—it removes the doubts from your mind. You know what your diagnosis is, and you are not self-diagnosing or assuming a diagnosis based on what you think your team is saying.

If the flu or a cold or any other contagious illness is flying through your family and you want to avoid it, tell your team what's happening. Nine times out of ten, they'll keep you from getting it. If it's unavoidable, your downtime will be shorter than it would be for those who don't use MAP and/or flower essences.

NOTE: If you become sick, I suggest that you have a MAP session daily. Among other things, the team can move you through the illness quickly. Your downtime will be much shorter. However, your symptoms may be more intense than you would normally experience. This is happening because the team is making sure your body processes the illness efficiently. Take essences, continue doing the MAP sessions, do what's needed to be comfortable—and blow your nose more often. You'll be out of the illness faster than you could imagine possible.

Consulting Other Health Care Professionals

I've written that you need to tell your team what therapists and physicians you are seeing. Then your team can work in conjunction with them. Also, it is good to open a MAP coning before you have your appointment. This way, your team can monitor what is being done for you. Then, as soon after the appointment as it is feasible, close the coning. Be sure you talk about the appointment in your next session so that your team will know how you feel you were affected.

If you see a chiropractor when you need adjustments, for example, your team will assume that you *prefer* to have your chiropractor make them. The MAP team will not override your decision to include someone else in your overall health team.

Although a MAP team is perfectly capable of doing chiropractic adjustments, they will not automatically do so in this situation. They will either tell you to see your chiropractor or assume you will see him on your own. If, from time to time, you want MAP to do the adjustment, you must specifically request it. There is no competition going on here. Your team will respect your preferences.

And finally, if you have been diagnosed with a serious illness, don't limit the scope of your treatment by ignoring alternative and quality allopathic options and just focusing on MAP. Let your team assist you in choosing the best combination of options the medical community can offer you. If you are battling a serious illness, you want to attack the problem from every angle and every level. The team concentrates its work in two areas: 1) it assists you and helps you coordinate the available options as you seek to put together the best possible treatment program, and 2) it works directly on your body, emotions, mind, and soul in conjunction with the full treatment program and in ways that are unique to MAP. In short, by including MAP as a major part of your treatment program, you will ensure greater efficiency and effectiveness as you work to reclaim your health.

Emotional Therapy and MAP

I think the best way to get across the value of working with MAP for emotional issues or while you are working with a therapist is to let people who have had this experience describe it.

My therapist thinks I'm a whiz kid at psychotherapy. She can't understand how I so rapidly moved through my therapy and so quickly brought needed changes into my life and began using them. Little did she know that I did a MAP session before each therapy session and fairly often another MAP session afterwards. I'm sure with MAP plus flower essences I got through it in one-third the normal time.

In therapy I have come to see how I survived my childhood by parenting my parents. I learned to disengage the active, powerful, intelligent parts of myself so that I could maximize the supportive, nonthreatening, nonquestioning side of my nature and be the dependent child they needed. Even though I've progressed quickly with this issue, when I'm with my parents the same

100

"dismembering" of myself still occurs if I'm not watching carefully—right before my eyes.

During a recent visit, at the time of my son's graduation, when I needed to be functioning well, this began to happen. I escaped to the bathroom and opened a MAP session. I explained exactly how I was feeling; I said I was feeling very afraid because I had incapacitated myself to protect my parents, but that this left me feeling helpless and insecure and, of course, angry. I was afraid that my insecurity would lead me to hurt them and spoil the occasion.

Lying on the floor of the bathroom, under a towel, a change occurred. When I emerged, I was again in contact with myself—strong, together, fully functioning, no longer angry, and able to enjoy the rest of the visit. The hectic day went by very smoothly and was actually enjoyable for everyone. To me this was a major miracle.

M. B., Maryland

Being in a new relationship has brought up old issues for me around boundaries, violation, fear of abandonment, etc. MAP and I have moved entire patterns out of my body and psyche by stating my intent to let the pattern go and follow directions. I connected with the White Brotherhood "incest recovery unit"* and in half an hour moved out a pattern that had plagued me for years. The energy of violation left, as did three men who were inappropriately connected to my energy system. For several days, I felt like my "clothes" were too big for me. There was so much *space* in my body. And, when making love, it was *my* energy only in my body for the first time.

Also, I've also had a big destructive "fear of abandonment" pattern come up in response to my partner's healthy need for more time and space to himself and less frequent sexual encounters—finding the balance. So we did a coning and I was told I was using sex as the antidote to fear of abandonment and what

I really needed was to anchor the pattern of unconditional love. So, one by one, I went through every relationship where I'd felt rejected and abandoned, forgave that person, asked for forgiveness, and experienced unconditional love. It took several days of essences to stabilize this work. I have a whole new outlook on how my partner and I use our time together and apart, and it is wonderful!

M. L., Ohio

*For doing specialized work such as incest recovery, simply connect with your MAP team in the usual way, inform them what special situation you would like to work on, and request that you have the appropriate members on your team for this work. This may be a modification of your personal MAP team, and you need not have a separate code name or symbol for them. Just connect with them within a regular MAP session by making the above request.

I had returned from an out-of-state funeral for a friend of mine. He was a young man with a wife and four small kids. He died in a totally unexpected and tragic way. It was a full military funeral. My being around the grieving relatives and friends, and the ceremony affected me deeply. I had been sad about it before, but when I got home it was as if I had picked up the grief of everybody and brought it all home. It felt as if it were impregnating my uniform and clothes. I felt a hollowness inside. I felt emotionally stunned. I couldn't concentrate and get on with my life. So I had a MAP session and asked for help in getting past that. As soon as the session was over, I felt totally cleared. I still felt sad at losing my friend, but I was free of that smothering cloud of grief and my life was back on track. This felt like a miracle.

E. R., Oregon

Flower Essences, Kinesiology, and Herbs

FLOWER ESSENCES: I've said that it is not necessary to include flower essences when doing MAP. And I certainly wouldn't want anyone to shy away from MAP because they feel learning how to use flower essences would just complicate matters. However, at MAP workshops I have asked people who began the program without using the essences and then included them later, if the essences made a difference. Only once did someone say no. Everyone else talked about how much clearer the sessions were for them once they incorporated the essences. They also talked about how much more efficiently and quickly they were able to feel the results of the sessions. And many said their ability to hear and sense their team improved tremendously. I thought I would just give you this little nudge if you are thinking about this issue.

In Appendix C, I have listed the steps for the three main flower essence testing processes that can be used with MAP: the basic test, the surrogate test, and the telegraph test. For further information on flower essence testing, I recommend the book *Flower Essences*.

Some people have tried to get around the issue of learning to use flower essences by emptying all the essence bottles in their sets into one jug, and taking a swig of this at regular intervals. Ahhhh—nice try. This only complicates matters. By taking all the essences at once, you require your body to cast off the ones that aren't needed. This is what the body does naturally with essences that aren't needed. You are now putting an additional burden on yourself. Plus, by taking a sip from the all-purpose jug, you don't know which essences you actually need, and you don't have any input as to how you are reacting and responding both to the work and to the specific issues that are being worked on. You have eliminated a useful feedback tool.

To clarify: You test for flower essences after you open a MAP coning and at the end of the session after you close the coning. You also test during a session when your team tells you to test or when you are going through a bit of a rough spot.

KINESIOLOGY: Like flower essences, you do not need to know how to do kinesiology to do MAP. However, as you develop your relationship with your team and the work, you will most likely want to ask specific questions about different issues. Kinesiology gives you the ability to bridge to your team. You ask them a simple question in a yes/no format. They project the energy of a "yes" or "no" into your electrical system. You do the kinesiology test on your electrical system, and from this you discern if the team's answer was "yes" or "no."

As I mentioned earlier, if you are overwhelmed at the idea of learning kinesiology or you are having problems with it, bring it up to your team and ask them to help you over the hurdles. You'll be surprised how fast you can learn to test!

HERBS: Many people who are attracted to MAP have already incorporated other alternative systems into their health care program. One system is herbology, the use of herbs and herbal extracts. Herbology comes with a large body of information that has been passed down through the generations about how to use herbs and which herbs can help certain problems. If you already use herbs in your health care regime, and are interested in using them as part of MAP, you will need to approach herbs differently.

MAP uses herbs in new ways. It's quite a departure from the traditional understanding of herbs. The easiest way to describe the new process is to tell you to test for them as you would flower essences. In a session, ask your team if they would like you to take herbs either generally or for a specific problem. If you get a "yes" (audibly or with kinesiology), then kinesiology test the herbs you have available. If nothing tests positive, ask if you need another herb. If so, test a list of herbs. An order form from the herb company you deal with will do the trick. Or make a list of the herbs your local health store has available, and test this list. Whatever herbs test positive are the ones you need.

If you need several, ask if you are to take them as a unit or separately. If they are to be taken separately, find out the order they are to be taken in and how many days/how many times a day you are to take each.

See Appendix C for how flower essences are tested and how dosages are discerned. Use the same concept and procedure when testing for herbs.

In short, by getting your herbal information through MAP, you are finding out from your team which herbs will work best for you for a specific situation rather than relying on the common, possibly outdated herbal information that may not apply to you at present.

Those people who have studied herbology and worked with herbs for years, and who then allowed their teams to prescribe for them, have said that they were amazed at how much more efficient and useful the herbs were with MAP. They also said they were surprised—sometimes stunned—at what herbs they were "told" to use.

Helpful MAP Aids

KEEPING NOTES: Take notes on the sessions. Record the difficulties and problems you talked about, sensations you felt during the session, and results you perceived after the session. At some point down the road, these notes often reveal patterns we had no idea existed. They also help confirm to *ourselves* that something really is happening in MAP, that it's not our imagination. And sometimes we go into a period of MAP work when we feel *nothing* during the sessions. We swear nothing is happening. We even entertain the notion that perhaps our team has walked out on us! But it's just that the work they are doing is, for the time being, on levels we can't perceive physically. Everyone in MAP experiences this at some point. When it happens, just continue with your session schedule. At some point, the team work will shift and you will once again feel things during the sessions. In the meantime, a casual review of the notes reminds us that, indeed, these sessions are for real.

PERELANDRA MAP WORKSHOP TAPES: We have available the tapes of the latest MAP Workshop that was held at Perelandra. Many questions are answered and many valuable things were said by folks who have been working with MAP. Quite a few people have told us that they found the tapes to be especially supportive. Ordering information is in the back of this book.

GROUP SUPPORT: When *MAP* was first published, folks told us that they wished they had someone to share their experiences with, but no one near them had ever heard of MAP—or wanted to hear of MAP. Now there are quite a few people using MAP, and it's not so hard to put together a support group.

We offer a special networking list for MAP people only. If you wish to be on the list, drop us a note and let us know. This makes your name and address available to others who are in your area and want to talk with someone about MAP. If you would like a list of people in your area who are on the networking list, send us a note about this, too. (You don't automatically get information about others in your area just by requesting to be put on the networking list.) We will send you the list.

The following is a newsletter article about one MAP support group. We titled the article "MAP Anonymous."

As a practicing registered nurse, I see a huge potential in MAP. Ultimately we are all responsible for our own health. MAP gives everyone easy and simple tools to do just that. Western medicine does not yet have a true understanding of who does most of the work concerning health and wellness. It truly is not the doctor or nurse, acupuncturist, herbologist, chiropractor, or massage therapist, etc. It is each of us individually. MAP provides us with the necessary knowledge. To work directly with MAP is quite a profound honor. Thank you for starting me on such a wonderful journey.

In January 1992, I received a surprise letter from another flower essence user in my area. She requested we get together for sharing and learning about MAP and flower essences. I had taught her childbirth several years before and had no idea she knew about essences. On February 9, 1992, we had our first gathering ... four women. All of us came with a wide range of life experiences, diverse educational backgrounds, and lifestyles. It was wonderful. We talked for hours. I'd like to share some of the common experiences we had while using MAP.

1. Since January and February of this year, a lot of us noticed strong sensations of pressure or pain/tenderness in the head area, frequently at meridian points or along the natural suture lines of the skull. Each of us was surprised at having similar symptoms at the same time!

2. During the early sessions, some of us saw an extraordinary green color, not previously seen. It was an almost fluorescent hue.

3. Each of us had been given what we felt was confirmation of our connection with nature during the early sessions. Our experiences were different and totally unexpected. As an example, immediately after my first session with MAP, as I opened my eyes, I saw brilliant, beautiful, green letters on the ceiling. I distinctly remember reading them one by one, as random letters. It wasn't until nearly an hour later that I realized the letters were P-A-N. The realization was quite profound.

4. Each of us had an awareness of MAP workers coming into our energy fields and leaving. Some members initially

experienced the exit of the team as quite abrupt and jarring, but not painful. When we requested that this be less abrupt and smoother, in the next session for each of us it was!

5. Each of us had a feeling at times of cold/shivering during the sessions.

6. Each of us had a pattern of essence use with MAP: lots of essences needed after a session, but next time a few. This was an alternating pattern.

7. Most of the group received verbal (audible) or intuitive help via conversations during MAP.

8. Some of us just experienced the physical presence of our MAP teams through sensations in our bodies.

9. All of us experienced complete relaxation and a feeling of wholeness during a session, and a desire not to end that session, or to have another session soon to experience that place again!

10. All of us have had nothing but positive, pleasant healing experiences using MAP.

Our small group tries to meet monthly to share experiences and gain reinforcement and encouragement regarding MAP.

We all seek the full understanding of who we are and how we can maintain, improve, or regain optimum health by using ourselves, and reaching into that all-powerful inner source.

Our families often ask about MAP. Some have been very receptive and are using the process. Others quietly observe and accept our choices without wanting to participate in any way... yet!

In all this, we are each learning our own inner truths, and gaining support and companionship from our group and our MAP teams. It helps to maintain a good sense of humor when we challenge ourselves with family strife, job uncertainty, parenting issues, or health problems. This support is reinforced for all of us at each gathering.

J. H., Massachusetts

A Note of Caution about
Sharing MAP with Others

IMPORTANT: Many people who have success with MAP suggest the book and the program to their friends. Please—Be sure that when you make the suggestion, you are prepared to share your copy of *MAP* with them. Or buy them their own copy to give them when you make the suggestion, if you don't want to let go of yours. Don't, under any circumstances, just give them the easy reference steps in Chapter 8. Worse yet, don't just tell them the steps. Everyone who gets into MAP needs to be fully informed. And they need the information to be unfiltered. This is so they can develop their own relationship with their team in a balanced and safe MAP enviroment.

One woman at a workshop said that whenever she gave someone a copy of *MAP*, she included the *Perelandra Garden Workbook*, as well. She felt the *Workbook* gave a valuable foundation for anyone working in MAP.

NOTE: MAP may be the best thing to have ever come along for you. Your life may have changed in dramatic and exciting ways since you started the work. Because of this, you may have a burning desire to share MAP with everyone you know—and maybe even some you don't know. I ask you to be sensitive when sharing MAP. If you don't know for sure that the other person would be comfortable with this information, be caring and considerate about sharing the information with them.

110

What Does Not Happen in a MAP Session

Some of these things I have already written. But I think they bear repeating.

You are in control of the coning at all times. The MAP teams do not open a coning on their own. *You* must do this. And the teams will not refuse to close down a coning. Once you indicate a coning is to be closed, it is closed. The teams will not ignore or override your requests. Also, your coning is perfectly protected. Nothing more needs to be done to "shore it up." However, someone who has paranoid tendencies or extreme victimization problems should not enter into the MAP program. They will not be able to accurately discern what is happening to them and will automatically turn MAP into a frightening experience. If such a thing is happening to you, stop using MAP immediately, and work on your personal issues in ways that don't set up an automatic fear response. No matter what, MAP cannot protect you from yourself.

MAP is a medical program. It is also a *human* medical program. MAP is not intended for animal care. (See Chapter 11 for the Nature Healing Coning for Animals.)

The MAP teams are not hoodlums. They do not kill your begonias or steal your money. Although you will experience love and respect from your team, they will not say things like you are the only one who can save the world—then proceed to give you a long list of wacky things to do for saving said world. These are all self-conjured experiences that spring out of fear or a

111

deep desire to "live a significant life." If you are having such experiences or are "hearing voices" that say strange things and won't stop, tell your team and let them help you regain your balance.

OTHER PEOPLE'S MAP EXPERIENCES

In 1989, I introduced MAP during a workshop. The folks were given the steps and encouraged to try the program. Several months later, I sent out a letter asking them for feedback as to whether they were working with MAP and what their experiences were. Out of fifty workshop participants, thirty responded that they were now working with MAP. They gave me permission to use portions of their letters so that others could benefit from their experiences and thoughts.

Several of the letters are from our newsletter. I'm including these because I feel they also say something that will both assist and support others.

I was not ready to do this kind of work for a long time. I respected that as an indication that the timing wasn't right for me yet. I also think I wasn't yet ready to make the commitment to go through whatever changes would be involved. However, during the past holidays, I began to feel that the time was right to begin. So, after checking with my higher self to make sure, I had my first session in January.

My scanning session seemed fairly uneventful. I had the sense nothing was happening yet, other than everybody getting acquainted. I did get my symbol when I asked. An image of a torch popped into my head as soon as I asked.

I have been doing the sessions twice weekly, but have just gone to a once-weekly schedule. My normal time to do them is about 8:00 P.M. I start by making the coning connection as you outlined. Then I ask if I need any essences and take them. I keep a notebook handy and record the essences and any issues and experiences that come out of the session. I do the sessions in bed, usually with a pillow under my legs.... I set a timer in the kitchen for 45 minutes, and then go into the bedroom. By the time I connect, test for essences, and get into bed, about 40 minutes are left for the session. Usually, I sense that the session is winding down a few minutes before the timer goes off. I thank everybody, close the coning, and retest for essences.

I have felt very little physically while in the sessions, including the initial scanning session. There has been no pain or unpleasantness so far, except for one session where I felt very restless and found it hard to be still.

I think the main issue we've been working on has been an emotional one, centered around my self-worth. Often, I start the session drifting off into sleep, only to awaken suddenly with some image or flash of insight, and a sense of clarity and light about who I am and what I'm doing here in this present life. It seems like maybe the drifting off is the way we have of getting my day-to-day mind out of the picture for a while so that the rest of my mind can say something to me. I do feel that the insights are coming from me, and that MAP is just facilitating the process.

I have had a couple of more physical experiences. Once, I felt embraced by a very warm and loving being, in an aura of total acceptance. It was an immediate kind of thing, not something airy-fairy. Another time, I felt like I was filled by a clear, bright light that made me buoyant. Both of these only lasted for seconds, but were so strong that the feelings lingered way past the session, and actually return whenever I remember them.

It took me a couple of sessions to get used to doing it, but now I make a point of verbalizing what issues I'm bringing into the sessions and what I'm experiencing during it. . . . Speaking makes things clearer to everyone involved.

The main word I have for how the MAP team works with me is "unobtrusive." I know they're there and I feel things happening, but it's subtle. It's like they take their cues from me and never force anything. The image I have is that exercise where two people face each other and one makes movements that the other duplicates, so that the first person feels like he's looking at his image in a mirror. It's that sensitive quality I feel from the team.

After almost two months of sessions, I have to say that MAP is very helpful and really pretty easy to do, once you make the commitment to do it. I have felt more clarity in my life and a greater sense of being connected with a larger reality. I credit MAP for some of the moves I'm making in my Feldenkrais work. I've found that MAP doesn't eliminate any issues or any work on my part but makes it all flow better. I have this image of the team squirting all the creaky, rusty joints of my being with oil to make them work smoothly.

C. W., Virginia

Yes, I have been using MAP; and, yes, it is a test of faith. I needed to address lingering issues of self-worth first—i.e., the belief that my life and work are not "important" enough in the universal scheme of things to "deserve" such specialized medical treatment. I knew from the moment they began surfacing that these thoughts were/are erroneous, but the more deeply anchored feelings accompanying them kept me from contacting the MAP and requesting their services. Working through these feelings eventually led me to realize the significance of the law of free will and also Jesus' statement "Ask and you shall receive."

K. W., Michigan

My basic issue centers around feeling comfortable with something that is beyond my five senses. I have experienced subtle body sensations, seen energy patterns swirling in front of my eyes, and gotten hunches that I should do things, but I still sometimes get angry at myself that I don't experience these sessions with greater conscious awareness.

Interestingly enough, in spite of not feeling competent about my ability to sense what's going on, the initial scanning session seemed very real to me. I needed essences to start the session. I got my team's name easily.... I saw something that I interpreted as my team's symbol (a swirling circle of energy that was also pulsating and contained a number of brilliant points of light or stars). I also felt some tingling in my arms and legs as if energy were being run through them.

C. P., Virginia

After I attended your workshop, I knew immediately that I had to work with MAP. The problem that I have hasn't been helped in 12 years with medical practice. The scanning session went well. I felt energy going up my spine and head area. At times I felt back pain, neck pain and was uncomfortable. I received no symbol.

During my first session, I spaced out several times. They were spinning my head around (a very strange experience!), worked on the cranium. Also they spun my hands around and worked on the hands. Then I was given a symbol.

Oddly enough, in the beginning I bought a little notebook and recorded everything in it. Alas, it came in handy.

I have no fear about this work, but then I perceive mostly through intuition. Sometimes I feel like an idiot lying there for 40 minutes talking to the air. At that point I'll say, "Please give me a sign you are there. I feel so dumb." And then I would feel someone brushing against my forehead or hair. Without doubt, I know that someone is there with me.

R. S., Pennsylvania

115

Scanning session: I was very excited and curious to start the process. . . . I felt a little awkward not knowing who or what I was talking to. I felt the presence of four—three males and one female. I asked if that was correct and received an affirmative. For most of the first session I just listened and "felt" what was happening. I did feel a lot of movement, pressure, all around me, especially around my head and abdomen. I would occasionally describe what I was feeling and ask if it was them. I would always receive an affirmative reply by "testing."

For the rest of the sessions, meaning up until now, I haven't perceived the presence of anyone but continue to feel the energy sensations—although at times it is so subtle that I sometimes wonder if it is all my imagination. Close to the end of the first month, I started asking for some kind of confirmation. That is when I started "dreaming" a *lot*.

The only consistent part of the sessions has been that no matter how hard I try, or the time of day or night of the sessions, *I always fall asleep* if for only the last few minutes. Then I will wake up only to find the session over. Re: how I have felt changes.

I "feel" that I am in some kind of "process" that I can't really articulate, but I feel comfortable and good about it. I feel a seriousness about the process—don't know if it's me reflecting back to me or if I am actually perceiving the team to be a really serious team. A little kidding around would be welcome—I think.

J. B., Virginia

Even though I was thrilled to receive the MAP technique at the workshop, it took me 2 or 3 weeks to get up enough nerve to start doing it.

The scanning session was interesting. I felt like I was being scanned by different energy sources in a very methodical way— from top to bottom and sideways. In my mind's eye, I "saw" different colors as the different scans were done. I also had

116

impressions of different large instruments being pointed at me. One was something like the projector used in a planetarium, sort of. My symbol is the sun....

My first session was quite unsettling. My father died in October after a long decline. What they had me do was deep breathing, then I became very nauseated and almost threw up, then I started to shout, "I hate my father." In fact, for the next week, I periodically said that, either in my head or out loud. During the whole time, I felt detached and kept thinking, "Isn't this interesting?" During the second session, I also did deep breathing to the point where I thought I was going to go into a re-birthing experience, but I didn't. Subsequent sessions have been much gentler at my request.

Since June I have been trying to get over thyroiditis, mainly working with my chiropractor to rebuild my immune system. I also practice the Radiance Technique.... I give myself a treatment every morning in bed before I get up. When I told my team about the Radiance, they said to set up the coning and give myself my treatment, and they would work "within the energy." So for about three to four weeks now I've been doing that. I also experimented doing it without MAP after a week to see if I could tell the difference, and I really can. The energy is amplified.... I don't talk out loud to them, only in my head. I don't "see" them physically or in my mind's eye, only feel their energy and sometimes, at the end of my treatment, I am filled with golden light and warmth.

M. L., Virginia

Scanning session: Felt light and floating most of the time. Sensation of energy around me and a bright light. Received symbol of "cactus." Now, when this first came to me, I immediately questioned it. I said to myself, "What? A cactus?" Then I just said, "accept it" and went on. The whole experience was very subtle, nothing dramatic.

Second session: During the day (before I did the second session) I felt very spacey, could not concentrate. I had pain in my stomach and abdominal area—seemed to be in the muscles running up and down and across my whole area. This sounds odd, but I had the feeling that my body, soul, and heart had regrouped, had pulled together. As if before, I had been sort of spread out and when I walked around I was dragging and catching on things. Now, I felt compact, strong, and more gathered in.

The pain cleared up about 30 minutes before I did the second session. After the session, I felt exhausted. It was hard to make notes and test for essences again. During the session I had no trouble talking with my team. I felt energy going through me again and again. I felt pain in my shoulders and back during the physical discussion. I had to swallow a lot and it seems like I was told to do that. I slept very deeply afterwards.

Third session: Was a very bright, positive session. Lots of energy, feeling of weightlessness very pronounced.

S. D., Pennsylvania

I started using MAP within a week of the workshop. Since I use the Energy Cleansing Process, I was comfortable in invoking the four participants in the MAP coning. I'm not a little awed and humbled at the generosity of the Deva of Healing, Pan, the WB Medical Team, and even my Higher Self, in making themselves so readily available.

I find it easy to talk with them and joke with them. For example, while I picture that they are working on me to help me physically accommodate spiritual expansion, I tell them that helping me relieve myself of some cellulite around my thighs would also be very welcome. I tell them about emotional issues I'm working on (e.g., resentment, aches and pains I've got, chronic tight sore throat, aching joints, how my eyesight is changing rapidly), what events are going on in my life (e.g., my kids both have a bad case of chicken pox, my spouse is living

118

across the continent with no plans for returning). I feel energy moving in my body during the sessions, particularly at the base of the spine and up my spinal cord. I also feel sensations in my neck, head, shoulders, pelvis, and the bottoms of my feet. It seems to me so far that the more I give them immediate feedback as to what I'm feeling, the faster the next sensations come. It's been pretty amazing, but never overwhelming. Frequently, I am relieved of aches and pains I had when I first lay down.

The biggest "problem" I have is finding the privacy and time for the sessions. (I'm essentially a single parent of an infant and a kindergartener, and I work and I'm 41 years old. Age gives me an edge on wisdom perhaps, but physically the child-rearing is harder.) I have even gotten a babysitter to have sessions.

What I feel overall from the sessions is that they are fine-tuning me physically and energetically, and I have an increased general sense of well-being. I feel emotionally nurtured from the sessions. And it seems they work very well with the other healing and spiritual work I am doing.

I've had a few sessions unlike the others. During the first two of the unusual sessions, I fell asleep—it was irresistible and I felt that it was okay with my WB team. I was jolted awake (a big, *soft* jolt) with a flash of white light in my chest. I pictured the team with the energy equivalent of one of those heart machines that are used to shock people's hearts into restarting. It was a surprising sensation, but not unpleasant.

The third session I want to tell you about felt like a non-event by contrast, at least initially. I wasn't aware of any sensations, energy moving, etc., as usual. I considered that I wasn't having a MAP session. As I lay there though, I realized that what I was labeling as "mental drifting" was much more vivid and meaningful than that. It felt like I was getting a lesson from my unconscious or right brain, and the pictures were in fact helping me to understand the issue I had asked my team to address at the beginning of the session. I don't know if MAP works that way (through pictures, insights, awake dreams) or not, but I feel I was getting some extra help from somewhere.

B. G., Florida

I find the sessions very enjoyable. The particular quality of awareness that comes during the sessions is unique in my experience. It is akin to certain experiences I've had from meditating and other practices, but has a distinct quality of its own. I usually feel a sense of expansion and peace that is wonderful and have found that the peace extends into my daily life more and more. This peace pervades the session—particularly during the first part of it. Even though I feel quite a few physical sensations during the sessions, some of them unpleasant, at the same time I feel quite detached from them. Toward the latter part of the session I often feel more "in the body" and the sensations are not as comfortable. I occasionally feel worse physically at the very end of the session but have found that the discomfort passes quickly once I become active....

I have made very specific requests as to what I want from the sessions and I have to say that these requests are being granted in a way that borders on the miraculous. I started out with some pretty major imbalances and am feeling that balance is coming quickly and profoundly. I started the Garden and Rose Essences a few weeks before I began the healing sessions and found that they started to help...and then these benefits accelerated dramatically once I began the MAP sessions. The combination has been extremely beneficial—bringing greater health, clarity, functionality, and peace of mind.

M. K., Virginia

MAP arrived "just in time." When I ordered it, I had no idea that I would need it. Yesterday I wondered when I would start the program. Today, I *knew*, and it was *now*.

Soon after entering into the session I became aware of an

almost weightless sensation and remember thinking "This is amazing. I expected to be one of those people who wouldn't feel anything and would have to go on faith." Then I had a strange sense of being turned, but not completely over. Soon after that, I was aware of an energy taking over my right hand and working with it. I figured this had to do with the trauma and consequent condition of my hand ever since my wrist was broken in 1985.

The next area my team worked on was my left hand. A month and a half ago, I told my chiropractor that I feared I was getting arthritis in my hand, and she examined it and said that a small bone was out of place. She corrected it and it improved at once. I hardly ever noticed anything with it anymore. My team worked on it for quite a while—longer than on any of the other areas.

At some point not too far into the session, I suddenly wondered what my symbol would be. Immediately "White Lightnin' " came to mind. That seemed inappropriate. "That can't be it," I thought. "I think that's one of the Rose Essences."

The areas I would have chosen for my team to work on, they did not choose. At least, to my knowledge they didn't. The second half of the session seemed uneventful, though I remained awake and alert. When the hour was up and I asked for my symbol, "White Lightnin' " came and nothing else. I was still doubtful, but said "Okay."

When I was writing the report of the session in my journal, it occurred to me to look up White Lightnin's definition. I was amazed and thankful, too. Suddenly, this symbol seemed perfect.

H. H., Pennsylvania

I'm a physician's assistant. A few months ago I reread your book *Behaving . . .* and then got on your mailing list. When I read about MAP, I knew I had to do it. I found *MAP* in a nearby bookstore, and this process has transformed my life more than I can describe. I want to tell you of some of my MAP experiences.

I was so excited when I found the *MAP* book that I read it in

121

one sitting and wanted to do everything immediately. It was the answer to my prayer in many ways. The next day I did the scanning session. I told them I was willing to give everything to this, I was ready to break out of my limitations, transform my life, and move as fast as I could while still being able to cope with my outside life. Man, they took my word for it! The scanning session was incredibly intense. After a few minutes, I felt I was being sedated, as if I were getting pre-operative medications given patients to make them groggy. I felt whooshes and rushes of energy in various places, and gentle probing and dissection, almost. I had very intense pain in one hip joint that gradually increased in intensity. I felt as if my bones were being remodeled. I didn't have problems with that hip before—just weird muscle spasms as a teenager. It was an exhausting and amazing experience. After the hour, I was drained and somewhat shaken— but had no doubts that this stuff was real! The pain in my hip continued for one more hour and then was suddenly gone. I thought, holy cow, if this was the scanning session, I don't know if I'll live through a therapeutic session! But for the next several days (I did it daily), the sessions were very gentle.

My sessions go through phases—lately I feel nothing at all, but there is a periodic humdinger. Sometimes I "blip out" through some or most of the session. At times I feel the most extraordinary sensations. Either energy or parts of my body are being scanned in grid works, as if they are being peeled off layer by layer, or just being touched. Sometimes I see things in my mind's eye, energy moving from place to place or funneling like tornadoes, or clear images of objects or places. Sometimes I feel the compassion, love, support, and enthusiasm of my team. This has made such a difference in my life. One of the greatest benefits to me is feeling I *do* have a team—a group of beings I can talk to and work with who care about me and help me. It eliminates a lot of the loneliness in life. I have studied and practiced many spiritual disciplines. But so many of them have such a gap between the inner experience and the outer life. With my MAP team, there is such a concrete, easy, and practical way to integrate *everything* in my life with my life purpose, deepest desires, and philosophy. Before this, I had felt so frustrated, stuck, and discouraged. I had hit a wall and didn't know how to get any further. Enter the MAP team! I don't have to know how. I just needed to be willing to change and do my best. And things have been changing, so easily and almost unnoticeably. From little things, like night-time foot cramps that I haven't had since I began the program, to seeing myself relating to people much more openly and freely, to my life once more being filled with happy coincidences and small miracles. I have seen changes happen on every level that I had assumed would take years of agonizing work.

Everything in my life isn't healed. I still have stuff to deal with, and new stuff comes up all the time. But now there is a way to actually work *through* it and not wallow in it for the next 20 years. Another change I see in my life is that I used to get sick when things began to be "too much." I'd get sick and it would give me an enforced reprieve and rest. Now when I start to feel myself getting sick, I can see why I'm doing it. Also, I choose to work with why I'm feeling overwhelmed instead of just taking a breather. And I'm not getting sick anymore. When I began the MAP sessions, my initial emphasis was on physical stuff, but very quickly the emphasis switched to basic issues like life purpose and my relation to the world.

E. R., Oregon

The following is from a physician who is using MAP.

This whole method of healing works on the electric/energy body level, I think, which then impacts on the physical over the next twenty-four hours. I can't think of a single thing it has to do with the allopathic medicine in which I was trained. However, I am a member of the American Holistic Medical Association, a group of physicians who are connected by their common desire to find a truer form of healing than the concept of the mechanistic (Newtonian) body, which we were taught in medical school. I think there are people in that organization who would be interested in this, and I am asking for guidance from my team on the proper place, time, and person for presenting this to that group.

I'm impressed that MAP is so easy—when I meditate it takes great effort and concentration to move my mind to "another place." With MAP I make the request, focus rather lightly on the coning and the team, and things just happen. Since it is a process that takes care of itself so easily, I think the most helpful thing for people to overcome fear and skepticism would be to read about others' experiences. I do know in my practice I have had to learn that some people do not want to be healed; similarly, MAP won't fit into everybody's needs or present state of growth. The beauty of it is, when one is ready, all one must do is ask for it. Truly a case of ask and you shall receive.

A. R., Arkansas

Chapter 5

The Calibration Process

In early 1990, nature came up with a brilliant process that is designed to balance us when we are having difficulty moving through times of emotional and mental stress. I began working with this process immediately and found that the Calibration Process can be easily combined with MAP sessions. And, although the Calibration Process is an excellent tool to be used on its own, I have found that the MAP/Calibration combination is even more effective.

First, let me introduce the Calibration Process to you as it was given to me in a nature session. Included are my comments about working with the process. Then I'll explain why it can and should be added to MAP and how you can do that.

SOME PERSONAL COMMENTS ON THE CALIBRATION PROCESS

I worked with this process extensively for nine months after I translated the Calibration Process session in March 1990. I wanted to understand and experience it before offering it to others, and I wanted to explore the different ways in which the process could be used. From the very first time I worked with it, I was amazed. I'd like to pass along to you some of my feelings about the process and give you ideas about when it can be used.

What impressed me first was the efficiency of the Calibration Process. It only takes a half-hour once you've explained the problem. Initially, I questioned this, not believing that so little time was needed to accomplish so much. In all of my work with the Calibration Process, the sessions have not exceeded the time it takes to express the problem and the half-hour. I'm quite used to nature coming up with exceptional co-creative processes that redefine the concepts of efficiency and effectiveness, but I was still impressed.

It took a little thinking on my part to figure out when I was in a situation that could be helped by the Calibration Process. It is *not* needed if we are moving through an emotional or mental process where we have a sense of forward motion being maintained. It's useful when we feel our wheels spinning or feel stuck and can't even begin to imagine how to proceed—in other words, when we're at a dead end. The Calibration Process doesn't sidestep emotional and mental processes. It is designed to keep our processes moving on all of our levels and "unjam" those places where we seem to have gotten stuck.

The first time I used the process was in March 1990, when I knew I was having difficulty addressing my work in the garden and maintaining focus on what I needed to do. I had tried every trick I knew that might "wake me up." I felt my ability to focus return, but it was short-lived, and I would quickly sink into what felt like a hole. I decided to try the Calibration Process. I set it up exactly as it was written in the session. I tried to explain as simply and succinctly as possible how I was feeling and how my life was being affected. And I admitted that I knew nothing else I could try. I sat for the half-hour and felt nothing happening. I closed the coning as instructed, assuming something would occur that would tip me off that I was now "healed" or whatever. Since I had done this session in the evening, I went about my "off hours" as usual. I still noticed nothing different by the time I went to bed. The next day, I began my day without thinking about either the process or possible changes. I just got on with what I had wanted to do. By the end of the day, it occurred to me that not only had I accomplished everything I could have hoped to do and more, but I had done all of this effortlessly. Not once did I feel I had to deliberately press myself through a project. I simply did it.

I wanted to share this first experience with you because it shows so clearly how the process can work without a bunch of bells and bugles sounding. In this instance, one day I was in one state of being (a difficult, unconstructive, wheel-spinning state) and the next day, after doing the process, I was in a completely different state of being. I didn't experience a linear progression from the first state to the next. I simply found myself there. Sometimes I have found in this process that there aren't any great and glorious moments of understanding and resolution. At times I have felt that the gears between my emotional and mental levels and my body are simply "off" and in need of a little calibration. So, nature gets everything back into sync, and the blocks that seem to cause the wheel-spinning unjam, and that's all it takes.

At other times, I did go through a resolution and understanding process that occurred either within the half-hour or within the twenty-four hours after the process. Again, it wasn't like some baseball bat hitting me in the head. Nothing that dramatic. I'd be moving along in my day and suddenly I'd know what the troublesome issue really was. Usually that in itself was the resolution. Or sometimes the resolution was in the form of action I needed to take to resolve the issue.

I have used the Calibration Process when I was mentally buzzing and couldn't stop, when I couldn't stop working, and when I could see that a fear I was experiencing was actually counterproductive and not helpful. Or, for some crazy reason, I found myself unable to make a decision even when I had all the information and input I needed.

Another example: When I give a workshop, I work with the Calibration Process in two ways. First, a week prior to the workshop, I ask to be calibrated for "workshop preparation" for the specific class. This puts me in a receptive, reflective, creative state, and helps me prepare the workshop in new and better ways. Second, twenty-four hours prior to giving the class, I have another calibration for what I call "workshop go." This calibration shifts me out of the more internal, reflective preparation state to the external presentation state. Their dynamics are very different, and I find that by using the Calibration Process, I am able to shift into both states with greater ease.

Everything I have experienced from this process verifies to me what nature says about the need to strike an involution/evolution balance within ourselves in order to function well—that is, working with nature and the soul as a team. All my calibration experiences have been accurate, efficient, and effective. In working with the process, I have grown and developed in the area of emotional/mental balance in ways that allow me to see more clearly new areas where this process could be useful. One of the first things I suggest to others as they learn about the process is to have a series of calibrations around the issue of understanding what constitutes emotional and mental situations that could benefit from calibration. I find that most of us limit our defintion of emotional to pain we experience in relationships and don't understand mental issues at all. I had to expand my own understanding before I realized that I could calibrate something like learning difficulties or persistent physical problems that have an overlay of mental and emotional issues I'm not aware of. Now if I suspect a Calibration Process would be helpful, I'll open the Healing Coning that is used for this process, and ask: "Is this a situation that could be helped with the Calibration Process?" So far, I've always been told yes.

UNDERSTANDING THE ISSUES HUMANS FACE AND WHY IT IS IMPERATIVE TO LINK IN CONSCIOUS PARTNERSHIPS WITH NATURE

It is becoming increasingly important for humans to understand the extensive partnership they have with nature, especially when focusing on issues of form and consciousness and all that this combination implies. We are in an interesting time in human development where the desires and needs of the human soul on Earth completely outstrip the ability of the present support frameworks. By this we mean support frameworks in all areas: agricultural, scientific, physical health, mental and emotional health, governmental, social, educational. . . . The development of the human soul collectively on Earth has surpassed the development of its support systems. In the nature-dominant environment that existed on the planet until the last fifty or so years, the human soul could more easily develop support systems that were compatible. One reason for this is that nature was abundant and could accommodate every human's needs. (We do not mean to imply that all needs were met, only that all needs could have been met had humans so chosen. The physical means for all human support could have been met at any time because of natural abundance.)

In the past fifty years, this balance has shifted and the planet has become human-dominant. Nature is no longer abundant enough to accommodate human needs and desires without careful consideration regarding the larger picture. We do not see this as a "bad" development. If ignored, however, it would be a dangerous development for all. But it is also a development that is forcing the human soul to expand on every level in order to address and survive the severe challenges that the shift to a human-dominant planet has created. Prior to this shift, individual human souls could expand and develop in ways that were not associated with survival. In short, there was a sense of leisure around this kind of expansion. The individual had a lifetime to expand his understanding from a broader perspective, while at the same time he devoted his efforts and energy primarily to those activities that served to support his day-to-day physical survival. Now, for the sake of survival on all levels, the human soul is required to make this shift, this expansion, and to do it quickly.

The present support systems were designed to best address human survival in a nature-dominant era that existed within a Piscean context (parent/child emphasis). Now the shift to a human-dominant era is being affected by the Aquarian impulses (partnership, balance, and teamwork emphasis). All of the previously workable support systems are crumbling. At the same time, humans are expanding. By this we mean that the human in the conscious state is expanding to enfold the human spirit in the unconscious state. With this fusion, when it occurs, the unconscious becomes conscious. Humans are beginning to understand in an immediate and personal way that life is far broader and more complex than they ever before understood. This expansion does not occur in a vacuum. It requires support on all PEMS levels (physical, emotional, mental, and spiritual) in order for it to be stabilized and maintained. So humans are expanding in their efforts to address serious survival issues on all levels, while at the same time they are having to function within a collection of frameworks that were never designed to meet the pressures of the present issues. There is an ever-expanding gap between today's expanding human and the planet's various social support systems' capabilities.

We have not gone off the topic of presenting the co-creative Calibration Process. We are giving you the background needed to understand the crux of the issues that humans face as well as why it is now so imperative for them to link in conscious partnership with nature in order to develop the support systems of the future—and we mean the near future!

The expansion of the human system requires that the expertise of nature in the areas of the relationship of five-senses form to energy and involution (bringing spirit and purpose into form) be tapped in direct proportion to the expansion. In your vernacular, the intensity and complexity of the game have increased to such a degree that the relative simplicity of the old support systems has been rendered ineffective. Humans must become partners with nature in order to establish the systems that will support the new complexity. Don't forget— the expansion of human consciousness to enfold its own unconsciousness includes the grounding of the entire expansion into form. Otherwise, the expansion will either falter or take on an ungrounded air and be useless. This expansion process is what is referred to as "the evolution dynamic." The grounding of the expansion and its expression through form is what is meant by "the involution dynamic." The human soul is being pressed to open beyond or soar above the existing support systems on the planet in order to see the new. To properly support this expansion, the development of systems enfolding the balance between the involution dynamic and the evolution dynamic is imperative.

And this is what nature can give you now. It understands the relationship of energy to five-senses form, and it knows what is required in order for the direction and purpose of spirit and soul to become perfectly seated into form in balance. As we have pointed out a number of times, nature is the master of involution and the expert in matters involving the relationship of energy to five-senses form. In order to create support systems that respond to this new demand of human souls seeking to ground a broader picture of reality into form, man must turn to nature.

We do not mean to imply that if man turns to nature for the needed development of his support systems that this development will be effortless or perfect. We have no intention of perpetuating a parent/child dynamic in our relationship with mankind. We have no intention of dictating structure and process. In fact, this would be impossible. Humans must supply intent, purpose, direction, and need when it comes to systems development. With this definition, we in nature will seek to supply the best structure in which to accommodate and move intent, purpose, direction, and need. It is a true partnership we seek. We will not interfere with or attempt to alter the human evolutionary thrust. We are here to assist and accommodate this thrust.

In medicine, humans have seen the relationship of nature to themselves in the areas of nutrition, natural medicines, and stress relief. Humans do not see themselves as nature/human soul systems requiring involution/evolution balance. Instead, *they see themselves as souls utilizing nature in form for the purpose of evolutionary growth. Nature has been the servant of the soul while the primary thrust of the human has been evolutionary. This cannot and does not work. The human system itself is a partnership between soul and nature, and its thrust, its primary focus, is the involution/evolution balance. When in form, and we mean by this any existence within the band of form, the human must strive for involution/evolution balance in order to achieve evolutionary movement. Without this balance, there is no evolutionary movement, activation, or change. The involution dynamic is the tool of the movement, activation, and changes required by the evolution dynamic.*

THE ARENA OF
EMOTIONAL/MENTAL HEALTH

First, let us say that we refer to this arena as "emotional/ mental" because the dynamics causing a person to be classified in need of emotional or mental assistance are, from nature's perspective, the same. The distinction between the two is created by humans and does not concern nature.

You will recall, Machaelle, from your personal exploration in this area that when you came upon an emotional block that seemed impossible for you to get through, you asked nature for help. We will say now that the insight to ask for help was, in fact, initiated from us (nature) and in response to our desire to assist you in anyway possible. You picked up on this insight and acted on it by opening a coning with the intent for us to assist you. It is essential that people understand that in areas where nature links with the human soul, it (nature) can only

134

do so on request. We do not assume a partnership. To do so would be to override human free will and thus render the soul powerless. This would be against universal law, and nature, on its own, does not live or function outside universal law.

As you told us what your emotional situation was, we observed the energy dynamics as they shifted and moved throughout your system on all PEMS levels. (We see the human system on all PEMS levels because that complete system is functioning in a form state.) We were able to observe the emotional blocks you were struggling with from the perspective of energy. From these observations, we were able to alter the blocks as well as the general movement of energy in a way that assisted and made more efficient that energy's movement. In short, we assisted you in achieving involution/ evolution balance in those areas where you had temporarily lost it. As a result, you experienced the shifts, insights, releases, and understanding required in the reestablishing of involution/evolution balance throughout your entire system. Remember, we see these blocks from the standpoint of energy—what is moving appropriately and what is not. We see your system as consciousness relating to form from the perspective of involution/evolution balance. We do not define what results in insight, understanding, and resolution. This is the evolutionary input for which **you** are responsible.

Our process with you is an example both of the partnership we seek with humans and how we can work together in every way to achieve full, inspirited, functioning form. Where the will of the human is present, and where we of nature have been requested to help, we will adjust, shift and facilitate the involution systems in order to support the human's evolution

135

process. For us, it is a relatively simple matter to work with you in this way. In fact, it is solely a matter of receiving a person's request for our assistance.

We suggest that we work together using the following process.

CALIBRATION PROCESS STEPS

1. Open a Healing Coning: Deva of Healing, Pan, a link with the White Brotherhood (state that you would like the appropriate link with the White Brotherhood for a Calibration Process), and your higher self.

NOTE: We recommend that flower essences be used in this process. We suggest that the person first test for essences after opening the coning and prior to stating the problem. This will stabilize the person throughout the process. A dosage need not be tested for, since any essences needed in the beginning of the process will be for short-term stabilization.

2. Request assistance with a problem on the emotional or mental level, or a problem on these two levels that is connected and physically manifested.

3. State the problem. State it as if you were telling a therapist. Talk about the problem itself and how it is affecting you physically, emotionally, mentally, and/or spiritually.

4. Once you have given a full description, allow yourself a half-hour to move through the stages of insight, release, understanding, and resolution.

NOTE: You may not perceive any changes in attitude or understanding during the half-hour. This will be because the *process of shifting understanding and changes in attitude sometimes needs to move through more complex levels in order to reach a point where one can perceive the effects. We suggest that if you sit quietly for a half-hour and no sense of understanding or resolution has come to you, simply move forward in faith that very shortly, within twenty-four hours, you will experience understanding, change, and resolution.*

5. We suggest that you test for flower essences again just prior to closing the coning and include a dosage/solution test for continued support during the post-calibration integration period. [In the MAP/Calibration Process, you'll notice that you test for essences just *after* closing the coning.]

6. Close the coning by asking to be disconnected from each member of the coning, one at a time. Test, using kinesiology, to make sure the coning is closed. (If you test negative after asking if it is closed, just refocus on the coning and again request to be disconnected from each member, one at a time. You simply lost your focus the first time. After the second time, you will test positive.)

ADDITIONAL NOTES: *We see some emotional/mental problems as comparatively complex layers of energy movement. It is quite possible that for the **final** resolution of an emotional/mental issue, one will need to go through this process several times—that is, a calibration **series**. As you move through the series, you will receive one insight after another. Each will serve as a building block for the foundation that is needed for the final overall resolution. But we stress that timing is a key factor. If and when a follow-up session is*

*needed, you will sense something related to the original prob-
lem that has become an issue. One need not plan ahead for
these follow-ups, for you will need time between sessions to
integrate the insight, release, understanding, and resolution
from the previous session. As you move through this for each
session, one layer of the problem will be eliminated or resolved
and the next layer will surface, and new questions or issues
will come up. Have another calibration session as the new
questions/issues are raised.*

*In these more complex situations, you will be moving
through a series of sessions with us that will resemble the
peeling process or two-week process described in the book
Flower Essences. As we have said, you will move through
one layer at a time, experiencing a sense of resolution after
each layer, which, once integrated, will signal you to move on
to the next layer.*

*The half-hour timing more than covers the time span we
need to move the human system through involution/evolution
imbalance into involution/evolution balance.*

*For twenty-four hours after a calibration, you may feel tired
and a little quiet—you may even feel an ache or pain that has
seemingly popped up from nowhere. These are simply reactions to the calibration and should be gone within twenty-four
hours. The flower essences solution from the post-calibration
integration-period will assist and stabilize you greatly through
this twenty-four-hour period. However, if a reaction should
persist, set up another Calibration Process around the same
issue and explain all of the various reactions you are having.
Nature will do additional adjustments that will either move
you through or eliminate the reactions.*

The Calibration Process is an additional nature-partnership procedure that is not in and of itself strictly a flower essence process. With or without the essences, this process can work. Flower essences would be most helpful, however, in stabilizing you throughout the Calibration Process itself and afterwards during the time needed for integrating the work accomplished during the process.

COMBINING CALIBRATION WITH MAP

The Calibration Process stands on its own and does not need to be combined with MAP. To do a Calibration Process on its own, simply follow the steps as outlined in the session above. However, for those who wish to work with MAP or are already working with it, it is more efficient to combine the two processes. By pointing out the differences in the two processes, I think you will more easily see why they are both complementary and advantageous for us to use.

When we are in a MAP session, we are in a coning that links us to our medical team and stabilizes that link throughout the entire session. Nature is a part of that coning and is essential in maintaining the link and stabilization while the team works with us. The work is done primarily between us and our White Brotherhood Medical Team.

In a Calibration Process, nature becomes an active team member in addition to its linking and stabilizing role. Nature, through Pan, shifts and adjusts us *physically* into an alignment that enhances and facilitates emotional and mental process. When we think about it, emotional and mental process is linked with every challenge we face.

When I am in a MAP session with which I am combining the Calibration Process, I feel as if my medical team is working with me on one level and Pan is in a closer, more physical proximity to me, working *in concert* with the medical team to move me physically through the session. The work done in a MAP session is efficient beyond belief. But what is accomplished in a combination MAP/Calibration session takes efficiency to the point of an art form. The White Brotherhood Medical Unit loves and truly appreciates working with nature in such a direct way. Because of their deference to our timing, they cannot initiate this combination for us. We must take responsibility for expanding MAP sessions to include nature in a direct, working partnership with us and the MAP team. Now it is rare that I have a MAP session without setting up a calibration in it. I automatically set it up to include the two just in case there is a calibration opportunity that arises during the session. I ask Pan, after setting up and prior to beginning the work, to do any calibrations that are related to the work going on by the MAP team.

I suggest that you try the Calibration Process on its own for a few times just to get used to how it feels. Then, combine it with the MAP sessions. But don't forget how efficient the Calibration Process is by itself. There will be times when you will know that you do not need a full MAP/Calibration session. You need only the Calibration Process.

Here's how to include the Calibration Process with MAP.

1. Open the MAP session as usual, activating the MAP coning. Test yourself for essences if they are part of your program.

2. State:
   I'd like also to open to Pan for the Calibration
   Process. I'd like that connection to occur now.
Wait five to ten seconds for this connection. Pan, who is already part of the MAP coning, will shift from that coning dynamic and move into a connection with you that is appropriate for the Calibration Process. You may or may not feel this shift. It is unimportant either way. If you use kinesiology, you can verify your connection with Pan for Calibration.

3. Now, explain to both your team and Pan what your difficulty is. You will be working together in a three-level team: you, Pan, and the White Brotherhood Medical Team. Continue through the MAP session as you normally would. Allow the session to last the full forty minutes.

4. When the session is complete, thank everyone and close down the coning. You will disconnect from:
   Overlighting Deva of Healing
   Pan *from within the Calibration Process link*

Pan *from within the coning*
Your White Brotherhood medical team
Your higher self

5. Test yourself for essences and dosage. (In MAP/Calibration, you test *after* the coning is closed. In a regular Calibration Process, you test just *before* closing the coning.) This solution will stabilize both the MAP work and the Calibration. Spend a few minutes quietly before going on with your day.

OTHER PEOPLE'S EXPERIENCES WITH MAP/CALIBRATION

I have always been interested in psychic phenomenon and have never experienced such, except dowsing. It is, therefore, with some incredulity that I experience the results after using the MAP/Calibration Process. Not only do the things that seem to be getting in my way get resolved, but often there is an accompanying insight. An incredible tool!! Thanks a thousand times!

R. L., California

The following is about using MAP/Calibration when we have physical problems and have also spent a lot of effort and time in trying to find the answers for eliminating them. When we have cast about in search of an answer that seems to always be out of our reach, this can add mental and emotional issues that then function as blocks to the healing process—anger, frustration, disappointment, depression. The Calibration Process addresses the emotional and mental blocks.

I began using MAP/Calibration and the flower essences about six weeks ago. My attitude to the processes can best be described by that old Biblical statement "Lord, I believe—help thou my disbelief." My mind was open but my faith marginal. Over the past weeks, my belief is gaining ascendancy over disbelief.

I presented the MAP/Calibration team with a chronic (12 years or so) neck stiffness, a source of ongoing discomfort, and frequent headaches. I had previously sought relief by a host of modalities including chiropractic, yoga, relaxation, and visualization exercises—and resorted mostly to aspirin.

After two weeks of MAP/Calibration and flower essences, the neck stiffness was much improved. Now it is gone.

A. G., Pennsylvania

Here's another suggestion for using the Calibration Process from an article written for our newsletter.

THE GROUP CALIBRATION PROCESS
by Clarence Wright

The Greek philosopher Heraclitus once said, "You can't step into the same stream twice." That wise philosopher used the stream as a metaphor for ever-changing life. Forms and structures never stay the same. Things occur; stuff happens. Just when we think we know the rules of the game, the whistle blows and the rules change. If Heraclitus were alive today, he'd probably be struck by how fast today's streams move.

Even though change is necessary for the evolvement of new and better forms, it sure can throw us for a loop. Today, rapid change occurs in businesses and other organizations where people work together for a common purpose. To be effective, organizations need to enfold new energies and constantly recreate themselves. What we're talking about is a change of form to more effectively meet the organization's current needs.

I'd like to share with you the Group Calibration Process we use at Perelandra to deal with changes in our form in two areas: integrating new employees into the organization and helping all of us work more in sync with each other and with Perelandra's overall purpose. Like other organizations, we are undergoing much growth and change. While this is exhilarating, it can at times stress us out and leave us scratching our heads and wondering what we are doing. The Group Calibration Process has been invaluable in creating an atmosphere of mutual support so that everyone can contribute fully to the work being done. It has been a great help in keeping us focused on *why* we do what we do, as *what* we do changes. It also makes available to us the assistance of nature, the acknowledged expert in form change.

The Calibration Process is a way of directly involving nature in change and making it maximally effective. It oils the gears and adjusts the screws to keep us from jamming up when undergoing change. What I would like to explain is how we use the process in a group setting and what it has meant to us. Any group whose members desire to work in a co-creative manner should find it helpful.

One person acts as facilitator for the group and leads everyone through the following steps of the Group Calibration Process.

1. If flower essences are available, all individuals in the group check themselves to see if they need essences for general balancing before starting. Those who don't know how to test themselves (by kinesiology or some other method of self-testing) can be tested by someone who does.

2. The facilitator opens a Group Calibration Process coning. The points of this coning are (a) the Deva of the organization, or group, (b) Pan, (c) the appropriate connection with White Brotherhood for a Group Calibration Process, and (d) the higher self of each individual doing the calibration. After the coning is

opened, each person checks again to see if he needs essences. Since the coning creates a new, temporary energy field around all those present, it's possible that a person may need an essence or two to help adjust to that new energy.

3. The facilitator states the purpose of the calibration, such as bringing a new member into the group or the group's expansion into a new area of work, or the group's need to work more cohesively as a team.

4. The floor is opened to anyone with thoughts or suggestions about what related areas the calibration should address. It's important that everyone be clear about the purpose of the session. It is also important that each group calibration cover just one issue. If more than one issue needs to be addressed, plan for a series of calibrations.

5. Everyone then sits quietly for about 20 minutes, or until the facilitator tests that the session is complete. The facilitator can tell when people feel it is over by noticing increased fidgeting and moving around. At the end of the quiet period, the floor is then opened again for people's impressions, thoughts, images, etc. This is where we have gotten some of our most useful information about what current changes will mean for our group. Sometimes people come up with similar images.

6. At this point everyone checks themselves for essences again, focusing on which essences would be helpful in grounding the information that came up during the calibration. Each person should check to see if an essence solution and dosage is called for.

7. Finally, the facilitator closes the coning, expressing thanks to each of the elements that made up the coning. Once again, each person should check to see if essences are needed now that the energy of the coning is gone. Dosage solution does not need to be tested at this point.

There is an eighth step that I highly recommend. Finish the meeting with some great chocolate cake or a fabulous lunch, topped off with espresso or a pot of tea. For us, this inspires some great sharing about the calibration in a very relaxed atmosphere. Be sure to have someone keep notes on the main points that come up.

The Group Calibration Process works so well because it focuses everyone's attention on the issue at hand. With nature's help in the process, people notice how grounded and solid the information is that comes out of the session. After all, nature is the master of grounding. And the best thing is that nature doesn't charge a red cent for the service! It's free for the asking. (Be sure to make your financial officer aware of this last point!) Also, nature makes house calls at *any* time, twenty-four hours a day.

Chapter 6

Emergency
MAP Procedure

Use this procedure for severe trauma caused by accidental injury, sudden severe illness, or sudden emotional trauma. I suggest that you practice opening this coning and "working" the process several times until you are comfortable and confident that you can do this in an emergency. Just be sure to let your team know you are going to do a few practice drills. It's best to memorize the steps, since you will not want to be rummaging around looking for them in the book when you're in an emergency situation.

You will be working with your personal MAP team. Obviously, then, to use the Emergency MAP Procedure you will need to already be in the MAP program and have a team.

TO OPEN THE EMERGENCY CONING: Simply state that you want to open an *Emergency MAP coning with the _____ team*. (Insert the code name of your team.) It is important to open the Emergency MAP coning *and* connect with your personal MAP team. The coning includes nature's stabilization, and the code name immediately links you to your MAP team. No special focusing is needed to open an emergency MAP session. Just make the above request (aloud or silently), and it will automatically happen. There is no need to verify this connection with kinesiology. This is a special setup designed to be used in serious situations when you can't afford the time it takes to open a regular MAP coning, and you can't focus on anything but your emergency situation anyway.

Once you are connected with the coning and your team (which occurs immediately), proceed as follows:

1. Take one dropperful of the pre-mixed Emergency Trauma Solution (ETS) every three to five minutes for the first twenty minutes after the trauma occurs. (Instructions on how to prepare this solution are given on page 155. The solution should be made as soon as possible and kept for emergencies.)

2. If you are able, immediately after this twenty-minute period, test yourself for flower essences for the injury or illness. Assume that you need these essences every thirty to forty minutes for the next two to three hours. (Prepare a solution bottle to take with you to the hospital, if necessary.) If you cannot do this testing, don't worry about it, and just get yourself to a hospital. Your team has been working to stabilize you from the moment you opened the coning.

3. Stay connected to the Emergency MAP coning and team during the trip to the hospital, in the emergency

room and for however long you are hospitalized. The Emergency MAP coning will support both your needs and the hospital treatment throughout this entire period. You need not do anything special to ensure that this is being done.

NOTE: If you are hospitalized overnight or for an extended period, test yourself for flower essences each day, if possible. (Refer to *Flower Essences*, Chapter 8, on testing during serious illness or injury.)

4. Once you return home and before you close the Emergency MAP coning, ask your team how often you should do follow-up MAP sessions for the illness or injury. This may be daily, weekly, every two weeks— whatever is needed to move you through a complete recuperation. If you are too exhausted or weak to open a regular MAP session according to the schedule your team advised, request that the Emergency MAP coning remain open for a few more days. By then, you should have the energy to open and close the regular MAP sessions, and you can close the Emergency MAP coning.

It would be good to do the regular MAP session as soon as possible. The physical energy needed to sustain an open coning will then be used in the healing and recuperation process. But in an emergency, the benefit that results from maintaining connection with the Emergency MAP coning and your team is more important than the energy you expend to keep the Emergency MAP coning open. However, during the normal recuperation period, this energy loss exceeds what is needed. In short, a continuous open coning is overkill.

While the Emergency MAP coning is open, you may talk to your team at any time. If you react to medication or treatment, or become uncomfortable for any other reason, tell both your team and the hospital staff how you feel. If you don't have privacy, you do not need to speak out loud to communicate with your team. However, it may be easier for you to keep focused on what you say if you whisper. During an emergency, you have *two* medical teams working with you: the hospital team and the MAP team. Keep feeding information to both of them. If you are explaining something to your hospital team, your MAP team will automatically "hear" it. You do not have to repeat it to them. However, if you are suddenly hit with severe pain or discomfort, tell your MAP team while you are waiting for help from your hospital team. MAP will begin to work on you immediately before the other team arrives.

SURROGATING AN EMERGENCY MAP TEAM

Just because you know MAP is effective and the Emergency MAP Procedure is especially effective does not mean that you should run around opening an Emergency MAP coning for everyone in need. Each person has his own patterns in life. The MAP teams respect this and are very careful not to impose MAP on anyone who has not given his conscious consent. The least we can do is demonstrate the same respect for others' free will, timing, and patterns. So, be careful when surrogating an Emergency MAP team for someone.

NOTE: It is important that you be with the person you are surrogating. Do not attempt to surrogate an Emergency MAP Procedure long distance.

1. If you know someone who already has a MAP team and needs an Emergency MAP coning opened but is unable to do it, you may do it for him. Just state the name of the person, request that an Emergency MAP coning be opened and that he be connected to his team (using its code).

If the person is unable to give you his MAP team's code, request that a MAP coning be opened and that _____ (name of person) be connected to his team. This will take a little longer (about two minutes at the most) as opposed to an immediate response if the code name is used. The MAP team prefers that the code name be used so that no time—even two minutes—be lost.

If you know someone who is in trouble but does not have a MAP team, *you must obtain his permission to open an Emergency MAP coning.* If he is conscious, simply offer to help him in this way.

I suggest that you spend a little time before an emergency occurs thinking about how you might explain MAP and the Emergency MAP Procedure to someone without making them die of laughter. It takes some thought, but it can be done. Make it simple and to the point. After all, in an emergency you don't have time to get into a deep philosophical discussion about the fine points of MAP. It can be as simple as saying that you would like to link them with a White Brotherhood Medical Team, a group of knowledgeable souls that will assist in stabilizing them. The link is immediate and can help them through the trauma or emergency period. They need do nothing except give you permission to assist the hookup. Just by saying "White Brotherhood Medical Team" it will give the person enough information to consciously decide if he wishes you to proceed. If this kind of concept upsets the person, you don't want to get into the position of assuming what's best for this person and overriding his life patterns by trying to "sneak" him into MAP. You cannot sneak a person into MAP. The teams will catch you every time. They can read the intent of the person you'd like them to work on. Without an okay, the teams simply will not do anything, and they will wait for you to close the coning. If the person in the emergency says no, you need to back off. As I've said, it is his option to choose. IMPORTANT: Don't prejudge someone. If you would like to assist in connecting him with Emergency MAP, just give the person clear, straight-to-the-point information so that he can make a decision based on his own gut reaction.

If he is not conscious, you still need to obtain permission. Make physical contact with the person. For example, you can rest his hand on your arm or leg. Ask to be connected to his higher self. Do this by simply asking! ("I'd like to be connected to _____'s higher self.") This will occur in about five seconds. Test using

152

kinesiology to verify you are connected. Then quickly explain MAP and the Emergency MAP Procedure just as you would for a conscious person, and, in a simple yes/no format, ask if it is appropriate for you to open an Emergency MAP coning for him. Test using kinesiology. This will work because you are now connected electrically with the person, and although he can't speak to you, he can still hear you and respond to what you are saying. You'll read his response electrically through the use of kinesiology.

If you get a positive response, ask that an Emergency MAP coning be opened for _____ (name). MAP will take care of the rest. Once they are connected, you need to release your physical connection with the person and ask to be disconnected from his higher self. ("I'd like to be disconnected from _____'s higher self.")

2. If the person does not have an Emergency Trauma Solution, you can surrogate test for one for this specific emergency. Do a surrogate basic test to clear him, and give him the needed essences. (Essences may be administered to a person in a coma by putting a drop of each needed essence on the person's forehead.) Then do a telegraph test beginning with the following question as the point of focus: "What flower essences does _____ (name) need for this trauma?" Test the essences. Administer the solution every three to five minutes for the first twenty minutes. (Mix the essences in a glass of water to make frequent administering easy.)

3. After the initial twenty minutes, surrogate test for a flower essences solution for the illness or injury and administer this solution every thirty to forty minutes for the next two to three hours.

In an emergency, if you do not know the nature of the injury or illness (which is often the case), simply telegraph test for "whatever has occurred because of this accident or illness." This will create an "umbrella" solution that will address all the needs as a unit.

NOTE: Working in a hospital, especially in an emergency room, will make it challenging (at best) to do flower essences testing. The above steps are a guideline for during this period. How much you can do for yourself (if you are the one in trouble) or as a surrogate tester will greatly facilitate the body's dealing effectively with the emergency. The MAP team will also be administering flower essences, but like the regular MAP sessions, there is often a twenty-four-hour "lag time" between when the team administers the essences and when they fully impact the physical body. This eliminates the trauma stabilization that can occur within the first twenty minutes when taking the ETS. Obviously, in an emergency fast action is essential. This is why taking flower essences yourself or giving them to an injured or ill person is strongly recommended.

4. Once the person is home or out of the emergency situation, *you* close the coning for him. *Don't forget to do this.* You must be with the person when closing this

coning. Request that _____'s Emergency MAP coning now be closed.

At that point, if the person is interested in pursuing MAP, teach him how to do regular MAP sessions. (Giving him a copy of *MAP* would be helpful.) He will not have to do the scanning session since this was already done in the Emergency MAP coning. He will need to request a code name, however, to facilitate his personal MAP sessions.

MAKING AN ETS: EMERGENCY TRAUMA FLOWER ESSENCES SOLUTION

Because everyone responds differently to trauma, this solution needs to be tested for and made for each individual. A generic trauma solution is a shot in the dark. It is someone else's idea of how he or she thinks you *ought* to respond in an emergency. For full effectiveness, you need to test this for yourself or be properly surrogate tested.

Another issue is when to take the ETS. Many people define trauma as being hit by an eighteen-wheel truck. If they are hit by a motorcycle, this does not constitute a trauma to them. I think the easiest way to describe when you should take your ETS is when anything happens— usually something sudden—that causes you to gasp and become alarmed. This actually covers all accidents: scalding yourself with hot water, cutting a finger while preparing dinner, slipping or falling on ice, or receiving sudden and alarming news. These kinds of things shock our electrical systems, and even though they may not always require that we open the Emergency MAP coning, the effects of that shock can be dramatically reversed if you take the ETS as prescribed during that first twenty minutes. Once the shock is eliminated, the body can work efficiently to heal the problem in ways that will, many times, appear miraculous.

So, be sure you have a bottle of ETS every place in your life where you risk injury—the kitchen, bathroom, tool shop, and garden shed. Or if you are especially accident prone or have a risky job, just carry a small bottle of ETS in your pocket.

IMPORTANT: You should not wait for an emergency to make this solution. Make it now and preserve it in 100% brandy or vinegar so you will have it when you need it.

Here's what to do:

1. If you are doing MAP, during a regular MAP session, state that you wish to test flower essences for your Emergency Trauma Solution (ETS).

If you are not doing MAP but would like an ETS anyway, you can still test for one. However, you will need to know how to flower essence test. To get your ETS you will need to connect to your higher self. ("I'd like to be connected to my higher self.") State that you would like to test for an Emergency Trauma Solution. Being connected to your higher self allows you to receive your full range of patterns when you are faced with an emergency, no matter what the emergency. NOTE: When you are finished with the testing, be sure to release from this special connection you have with your higher self.) Now follow steps 2 through 5.

2. Do a basic test first and take any needed essences. Then state that you would like to test for your ETS. Test for essences as you ordinarily do. The only difference is that you are now telegraph testing for your ETS. (For more information on telegraph testing, see Appendix C.)

3. Check the combination of essences that test positive to be sure that all of these essences are to be included in the ETS. Again, this is the same procedure you use for preparing any flower essences solution.

4. Once you have all the essences you need, ask how many drops of each essence go into the solution. (See Appendix C regarding essence dosage.) You will have to know what size dropper bottle you will be using for your ETS so that you can test for the proper number of drops for that volume.

5. Add the drops to the clean solution dropper bottle and fill it with brandy or distilled white vinegar. This bottle may sit around for several years, so the solution must be well preserved.

HINT: Make *several* well-labeled ETS bottles and place them throughout the house (one on each floor), in your office, in your car, in your briefcase, or purse. . . . Have them readily accessible and easy to find. In an emergency, you don't want to have to hunt for these bottles.

6. Every year, retest to make sure your ETS hasn't changed. If you've made any big personal changes, chances are your solution will need to be updated. If you just "feel" that you need to check your solution, do it. Most likely you need to update it.

NOTE: *An ETS should be made for each member of the family.* If other members are also doing MAP, encourage them to prepare their solutions while in session. If you have small children in MAP, you can surrogate test while they are in session for the solutions they need. Be sure to label the ETS bottles clearly and with large lettering so that in an emergency it will be easy to discern which bottle belongs to the person in trouble.

If other members of the family are not in MAP, you have to connect with each member's higher self to prepare an ETS for him. *Before testing for someone else, do a basic essence test on yourself to make sure you are clear.* Make physical contact with the person and ask to be connected to the family member's higher self. Test to make sure you are connected. Do a basic test for them, and give them any needed essences. Then request the essences that person needs for his Emergency Trauma Solution. For this testing, you will be working solely with the person's higher self and not in a MAP coning. Follow steps 2 through 5 listed above. *IMPORTANT: Once you have completed the steps, disconnect physically and ask to be disconnected from that individual's higher self.*

ADDITIONAL NOTE: The ETS is to be taken only during the first twenty minutes immediately following an injury (severe or not), or a sudden severe illness or other trauma. After this period, you must focus on the individual injury or illness when testing for flower essences. (You may interpret "injury" to include emotional injury, as well.) The ETS addresses the *initial* shock, electrical damage, and trauma the body undergoes in the first twenty minutes. After twenty minutes, the effects of this initial trauma become integrated with the injuries themselves. However, if controlled, the injury or illness is not complicated by the effects of the initial shock and trauma. Healing and recuperation are then greatly facilitated.

USING MAP FOR SCHEDULED SURGERY OR DOCTOR'S APPOINTMENTS

You could say that the Emergency MAP Procedure is used for *unscheduled* surgery and doctor visits. However, MAP can assist scheduled surgery and treatment in your doctor's office, as well. For this, you don't need an Emergency MAP coning. Open a *regular* MAP coning prior to surgery or your doctor's appointment, tell the team what you are going to do and any concerns or fears you have. (Test for flower essences!) Allow the coning to remain open throughout the procedure. If the surgery requires hospitalization, keep the regular MAP coning open for the entire time and work with your team as outlined in steps 3 and 4 in the Emergency MAP Procedure. Close the coning once you have stabilized and have the energy to open regular MAP sessions that will go on throughout your recuperation. For doctor's

159

appointments, close the coning after you return home, then test yourself for flower essences and ask if your team wants to schedule follow-up sessions.

By including the MAP team during scheduled surgery or appointments, the team can observe what is being done, how you are reacting, and assist and stabilize you whenever needed. Also, if you include your team in these scheduled "events," you don't have to try to explain to them in a regular session what went on. They've already observed what went on. You only need to tell them how you feel about what went on. NOTE: MAP is really helpful during dental appointments!

OTHER PEOPLE'S EXPERIENCES WITH THE EMERGENCY MAP PROCEDURE

In early April of 1992, I had an accident involving a sauna stove which I fell against from a pretty good height. My meeting with the stove resulted in first and second degree burns, a pretty deep cut and abrasion on the left side of my back, and a good amount of pain and shock. My partner had the presence of mind to locate a ride to the emergency room. She also grabbed the kit of Perelandra essences on the way out the door. On the way to the hospital, I opened a MAP coning and asked for some special assistance, and my partner tested me for essences.

After opening the coning and taking the flower essences, I immediately felt better. I was able to stay conscious and focused during our trip to the hospital and during the question-and-answer session in the emergency room.

While we were waiting for the on-call doctor to show up, my partner continued to test me for essences. She did separate tests for the burn, the cut and abrasion, and the pain. She and our friend who drove us to the hospital remarked at how fast the burn seemed to be healing. The blisters were actually shrinking before their eyes, and the color of the skin around the cut was changing quite rapidly as well.

By the time the doctor showed up, an hour and a half later, the whole wound looked much better. The doctor cleansed and bandaged it and told me to see a surgeon in the morning about whether I would need skin grafts.

After arriving home, I tested and was told to keep the MAP coning open during the night. When I saw the doctor the next day, he was impressed at how well the burn looked. He said that it was well on its way to healing and would do so without any complications as long as we kept it clean. He also said that the wound would probably scab over in a few weeks, which would cause some pain and discomfort, but that would be normal.

He suggested that I get a tetanus shot. I do not like tetanus shots, but reasoned that it would be a good idea. Before getting the shot, I asked my MAP team to work with the tetanus and move whatever amount my body didn't need right on through. I encountered absolutely no pain or discomfort from this shot.

After the initial trauma passed, we began testing essences for different aspects of the wound—the large area that was burned, a smaller deeply bruised area, and two separate deep gashes. Each area required a different essence combination. I found that the essences that were needed for the deepest part of the wound related to the core issues that I have worked with healing throughout my life. As I healed physically, I found myself viewing my life differently, and was able to shift some very old limiting patterns. With this accident, I literally crashed and burned. Through feedback gained from the essences, I was able to rebuild my life in new and constructive ways.

All in all, I was told to keep the coning open for four straight days, which I did. Three days after the accident, I was able to travel on a plane for six hours. The wound healed without forming a scab. Within four weeks, I no longer needed to bandage the wound. And now, about four months later, there is just a faint scar to remind me of this MAP miracle. I am very thankful for the support that MAP and flower essences provided during this experience.

S. J., Alaska

Last summer, I seriously cut three fingers on my right hand while mowing the lawn. One was cut off completely at the top joint. As soon as it happened, I called for assistance from the Emergency MAP Team. I was told "Everything will be all right" and felt a deep calm. It was so reassuring that I had no problem driving myself to the hospital, and never went into shock.

When the doctor in the emergency room began surgery, I talked to the EMAT (Emergency Medical Assistance Team) again, and experienced the room flowing with a wonderful light energy. My friend holding my other hand and watching the surgery said a noticeable change came over the young and somewhat inexperienced doctor. His shaky hands became calm, and he smoothly stitched the fingertips of my three fingers back together. Throughout the surgery, I focused on bringing energy down through my crown to my heart. My friend was sending energy out into my right hand as it was being sutured. All the while, we both felt this tremendous loving presence that filled the room.

Now, seven months later, the fingers have healed nicely. I have had MAP sessions consistently throughout this period and have continued to ask for healing in these fingers. The doctor is extremely pleased at my progress. There are only a few things I can't do as well as I could before the injury, but these are also diminishing.

I am very grateful to the Emergency Medical Assistance Team and feel very blessed to have known about this magnificent assistance at that crucial time. I would like to see the word get out to all who are open to this valuable resource.

P. D., Maryland

Chapter 7

Surrogating MAP
for Children and Adults

MAP FOR CHILDREN

When I wrote the first edition of MAP, it was quite clear that the MAP teams wanted people to develop their personal relationship with the program before attempting to use it with children. After all, to work the program effectively with children, an adult must be present, supportive, and comfortable with using kinesiology and testing flower essences. In the first edition, we said:

Generally, children do not need the kind of intensive help that MAP offers. There are other means that can be utilized to get comprehensive help for them—for example, flower essences. This is a simple, efficient, and *extremely* effective tool for balancing and helping children. And it is something they can relate to and enjoy taking. Flower essences are not a mystery to them—they can see, feel, smell, and taste the essences. MAP sessions may be scary since the child will be sensing and feeling things he or she won't be able to relate to or understand.

The MAP teams still stand by this statement. The vast majority of "normal" childhood illnesses and injuries can be effectively helped with flower essences. Plus, children love all those little bottles, and they learn how to accurately test for essences with extraordinary grace and ease just by observing the adult testing.

However, if you have a child who has a chronic illness and the essence testing isn't working for you, or your child has a serious condition, is faced with an upcoming and potentially traumatic change, or has already gone through one, you might consider "putting" him or her into MAP.

To do this, you must be prepared to function as the child's support throughout the entire session. My first suggestion is that you do not attempt to activate MAP for a child until you have worked with MAP yourself for *at least five months*. You will need to remain with the child for the entire session and assist him throughout.

For some sessions, you will just be sitting there the entire forty minutes quietly focused on the child and the session. That is, you will be passively present. During these times, you are to remain present (this is *not* free time for knitting or writing letters or drawing). The team needs to be able to get your attention if they need you to essence test the child or touch him in a specific way for either comfort or stabilization. At other times, you will be actively present. This means you get to jump into action. You will need to surrogate test and administer the flower essences to the child. You will also have to know enough about the different sensations to be able to reassure and comfort the child if he becomes frightened. And you will need to be able to communicate directly with the MAP team, using either kinesiology or whatever other method you have developed with your team, in order to discern specifics that the team wishes to pass along as well as the child's session schedule.

A child's MAP team talks to the parent, not to the child, about medical treatment and specifics. It is advisable to take notes during each session. Record the questions you ask and their answers; the essences that are needed; any insights you receive; any changes in diet; any changes in sleep or play activity. Ask the team the same kinds of comprehensive questions you would want to ask a good, communicative pediatrician.

In short, in a child's MAP session, the adult functions in the same responsible role as when taking the child to a pediatrician. The adult is actively present, gives pertinent information, asks questions, and receives instructions from the pediatrician. The same things are done in a MAP session. In essence, you have to be confident enough about MAP to function as a competent, relaxed support person. *Under no circumstances should you activate MAP for a child unless you can meet these criteria.*

I would also like to point out that you should not activate MAP for a child unless you are the legal guardian of the child or have permission from that child's legal guardian. I don't mean to emphasize law here, but rather intent. Legal guardianship implies certain rights between an adult and a child that include the right to make this kind of decision for the child. When a child is young, the parents or guardians take responsibility for making all the decisions concerning that child's health care. This is an implied responsibility that goes along with the position. At a certain age—which is different for each child—the child begins to participate in these decisions. At whatever point you feel comfortable with the level of maturity of the child to have a say in his or her health care, this is also the time when a child is capable of saying whether they wish to participate in MAP.

There is the issue of when to allow the child to do MAP, without an adult present. I've heard parents say, rather proudly, that their child is doing MAP by age seven or age nine, or whatever. (Always, of course, the child is special or gifted.) It seems to me this becomes a point of pride or some kind of race with parents—like how early their child is potty trained, walking, speaking, and reading. A MAP session is not about competition, nor is it a classroom or day-care center. It is a legitimate medical experience. If you don't think your child is mature enough to decide when he needs to see a doctor, and you don't feel comfortable letting him go through a doctor's appointment alone, assume that it is not appropriate to allow the child to schedule and go through a MAP session alone. Give the child and the team the support that is needed so that the health issues can be properly addressed.

Luckily, the MAP teams aren't dumb. If they see that a child who is not capable of handling sessions alone yet has opened one without an adult present, the team will not get into any serious work with the child. So you don't have to panic around this issue and hide the MAP steps from him. Your child is safe. The team will stabilize and relax the child, then wait for him to close the coning. If the child just gets up and trundles on to another "toy," the team will automatically close the coning for him. (The teams do not give this "service" to adults. They feel it is important that a capable adult assume the responsibility for closing a MAP coning himself.)

If your child becomes ill or is facing something else that is out of his usual pattern, and he has worked with a MAP team alone, don't assume it is appropriate for him to have sessions alone for this particular situation. If you are concerned and you want the team to work effectively and efficiently on your child, take the session seriously and be present for support and any needed assistance.

There is another age issue around MAP and children. We are all somebody's child. (Unless you are an alien and were formed from pond scum.) Here's the scenario: You are fifty-nine years old. You have been doing MAP for a year. You have found it to be an amazing and outstanding tool. It has given you the leg up on health issues you have struggled with for the last forty years. You have a forty-year-old son with asthma—and the idiot smokes on top of it. You know MAP could help him. But he thinks you are crazy and would not be open to anything like MAP. It's all alternative crap to him. It is not ethical to try to sneak him into a MAP session without his *conscious* permission. You may be his parent, but he is an adult, and his rights supersede yours. You do not have the right, even as his parent, to interfere in this way. A MAP team will not participate in a sneak attack, no matter how well intentioned a parent may be.

There is one area of health where it is appropriate for a child to develop a personal, private relationship with their MAP team. This is the area of emotional health. Think. Normally it is not appropriate for a parent to be present during a child's session with his or her therapist or counselor. The same would be true in MAP. If a child is comfortable with MAP and wishes for such a therapeutic situation, some place to go to share his thoughts, pain, anger, fear, and sadness, this is an excellent solution. In this situation, it would be best if the child knew how to open the coning, test for essences, and close the coning.

If the child feels more comfortable with you opening and closing the coning, you may do so. Open a regular child's MAP coning (including your higher self), then leave the room to give the child privacy. After the forty-minute session, return and close the coning. Then test the child for essences. The child needs you to open and close the coning—therefore your higher self is an essential part of the coning. Your presence in the coning is reassuring and comforting—and is still needed.

NOTE: It is important that the child test for essences *and dosage* himself or be tested by an adult immediately after each session is closed. The essences will stabilize and support whatever went on in the session.

MAP STEPS FOR CHILDREN

THE SCANNING SESSION

1. a) Open the coning. A qualified parent or guardian with at least five-months personal experience with MAP can activate the coning for the initial scanning session.

You must include both your higher self *and* the child's higher self in the coning. The following is the coning for the children's MAP scanning session:

Overlighting Deva of Healing (Wait ten seconds.)
Pan (Wait ten seconds.)
White Brotherhood Medical Unit (Wait ten seconds.)
Your higher self (Wait ten seconds.)
The child's higher self (Wait ten seconds.)

Allow another ten to fifteen seconds for the team to adjust the coning appropriately to facilitate the scanning.

b) Inform the White Brotherhood that you are acting on behalf of this child.

The child can be asleep for the scanning session and all regular sessions. You may prefer this since it is easier to keep a sleeping child still! If possible, it would be best for the child to be lying on his back. But if this is not possible, the team will work around it. Do not hold the child in your arms or on your lap for the session.

c) If the child is asleep and is too old to be given essences on the forehead (explained later in this chapter), just test yourself for essences and take the ones that are needed. You do not need to test for dosage for yourself at this point. If the child is awake, test him for essences also and administer the ones that are needed. By testing

169

yourself for essences, you are ensuring that you are fully stabilzed in the coning. However, the teams do not want you to wake the child for this testing because the advantages to both the team and the parent of working with a sleeping child outweigh the advantages of this essence test.

2. Placing your two hands side by side, palms down and parallel to the reclining child about three inches above the body, "scan" the child's body system to the team. This differentiates your body energy from the child's and connects the team with the child's system. Do this by moving your hands in concert, starting from the top or crown of the head, and moving slowly down the body to the bottoms of the feet. As you move down the trunk, you will have to move your hands in concert to scan each arm and then each leg. The movement of your hands should be slow and steady. If you can "hear" the team, they may tell you to hold the scanning at certain spots along the way. Just stop your hands and hold them above the body until you get the go-ahead to start moving your hands again.

Artwork by Sandra Hirth

3. The first session will last one hour. For the scanning session, you do not need to verbalize any problems or issues the child is dealing with. This is a quiet session for you. At the end of the hour, *you* request that you be given the child's team symbol or code. You will use this code to open any future sessions for your child. If and when the child takes over his own sessions, he will also use this code.

4. Close down the session exactly as you would for yourself, only now you must disconnect your higher self *and* the child's higher self.

5. Check yourself for essences, just in case your being in this special coning threw your balance off. Take any needed essences. Also test for dosage. Then test the child for essences. To do this, physically touch your child. (This connects your two electrical systems.) Ask: "What essences does _____ (name) need to balance and stabilize this MAP session for him/her?" Then test the essences as you normally would, and check for dosage. (For more information on surrogate essence testing, see Appendix C. For information on administering flower essences to children, see page 177.)

THE REGULAR SESSION

Most parents prefer for their child to be asleep for the sessions. Try to position them on their back, if possible. If not, the team will work around the contortions, but they won't be able to work quite as efficiently.

1. a) Open a children's MAP coning using the child's team code. Don't forget to include your higher self in the coning. The children's MAP coning includes:

Overlighting Deva of Healing

Pan

White Brotherhood Medical Team (visualize team
    code)

Your higher self

Your child's higher self

Wait ten to fifteen seconds.

b) Test yourself for essences and take what is needed. Then, if essences can be administered, test the child and give what is needed. Do not test for dosage for you or the child at this point. This test makes sure you and the child are stabilized in the coning. However, as with the scanning session, don't wake the child to do this test. A sleeping child is still a major plus.

2. The regular sessions for a child are also forty minutes. Tell the team all the information you can think of about your child's health patterns and problems— physical, emotional, mental, and spiritual. Be as comprehensive in information you give this team about your child as you are with your own team. It might be helpful to write down specific points you don't want to forget before going into the session. At the end of forty minutes, ask for any information about treatment or changes. Then find out from the team when they wish to work with the child again. It won't be like the adult schedule. It will be less frequent, unless there is a

chronic, serious problem. I am not giving a prescribed schedule of sessions for children as I did for adults because it is assumed that any adult participating in a child's session will meet the criteria of being able to communicate with the team. This way, they will be able to get the schedule that is best for their child.

HINT: It is easier to keep your focus if you say something out loud. However, this does not mean you have to say it so loud that you will wake up the child. Whispering is fine.

3. Close down the coning and check both yourself and the child for flower essences and solution dosages.

ADDITIONAL INFORMATION

It is important that you not hold the child during the session because the mixing of the two sets of energy will be too much for the team to separate and discern well. However, if you must touch the child for essence testing during the session or hold the child if he should become frightened, you may do so. The team will stop the session until you are finished. The forty minutes does not include "comfort breaks." So be aware of how much time is taken and add this to the forty minutes.

Sometimes the team will ask you to touch or hold the child in a specific way. This stabilizes him during the session. The most common "hold" involves placing one hand under the back of the neck (the cervicals) and the other hand at the very base or bottom of the back, just at the tailbone. This hand is stabilizing the sacrum. They may request that you hold your hands in this position anywhere from five to twenty minutes. They don't want you to lift the child up to do this. They just want you to place or slide your hands to these two areas and hold them there. Also you may feel intuitively that you are to touch or hold something. Before jumping into action, check your intuition with the team, either verbally or with kinesiology. Make sure you understand where they want you to hold.

As I've already mentioned, be sure to keep good notes on all the questions asked in a session, any insights or information you are given by the team, session scheduling, essence dosages.... You'll be referring back to the notes a lot. Also, keep notes of questions you think about and want to ask in the next session.

Ask lots of questions, and don't be afraid to make them practical. Focus on what is needed to get your child through the illness or injury as efficiently and effectively as possible. If your child is sick, don't waste time by asking a bunch of questions about whether this is some karmic holdover from your child's lifetime as an alcoholic ice sculptor in ancient Iceland. If something like this is important, you'll get the insight from the team. You don't have to go digging for it. Instead, ask about diet, flower essences, herbs, number of days of bedrest needed, and anything else that's immediately practical and helpful that you can think of. If you are using herbs with the child, approach the testing as described in Chapter 4. Let the team prescribe the herbs needed and how they are to be used. Don't assume that the herbs will be used for your child as they have been for you.

As with adults, MAP is not opposed to your using over-the-counter medicines or prescription drugs, seeing doctors or going to the hospital for children. Sometimes working from both ends of the situation is the most efficient route. They may suggest something to you along these lines. If you aren't confident about hearing them, ask direct questions about the regular medical assistance that is available to you. And even if the team says a doctor's visit is not needed but you feel uncomfortable about this, then take the child to the doctor. Do what you need to do to feel comfortable.

When you take the child to the doctor, open the coning for his team and keep the coning open throughout the visit. This gives the team the information they need to appropriately support and assist what is happening. After the visit, ask the team when they would like their next "appointment" with the child, then close the coning and check for essences as you would a regular session for a child.

As the supporting adult, you will need to take responsibility for getting the schedule for any follow-up sessions and letting the team know during these sessions any changes you have observed in your child's condition or pattern of behavior. Include both positive and difficult changes. This lets the team know how the child is integrating their work. On the whole, you will need to do follow-up sessions for your child just as you would for yourself.

Do not put a child into MAP if that child is frightened of a concept like MAP or is easily frightened by life. This is not the program for that child, no matter how much MAP could help. It would be unfair and unnecessarily frightening for such a child to deal with MAP. Use flower essences in this case.

Some parents who regularly use MAP with their children have said to me that sometimes they will open the coning while their child is asleep but they "hear" or feel strongly that the child does not wish to be disturbed. Even though the child is asleep his higher self knows you just opened a MAP coning. Apparently this kid doesn't want a session right then or is busy. Do not override this. The parents who have talked about it say it is unmistakable—and often funny. They just say quietly "okay" and close the session. Sometime during the next night or two, they try again—and everything is fine. There's no resistance.

If your child needs a process like the Body/Soul Fusion Process, plan to do it while he is in a MAP session. This allows the team to support and assist the child as he moves through the process. Open the session, state your intention of doing the process, verify with the team that it is a good time to do the process, and then move through the steps as outlined. Doing it in MAP does not alter any of the steps. (The Body/Soul Fusion Process is explained in Perelandra Paper #4. See the order form in the back of the book.)

MAP/CALIBRATION FOR CHILDREN: You would use the MAP/Calibration combination for a child in the same kinds of situations you yourself would use it. Consider a MAP/Calibration session when your child is emotionally or mentally stuck, unable to move forward, or suffering from learning disabilities. First, however, try working with these problems by using flower essences. Really, the vast majority of these kinds of issues can be easily addressed with the essences. Children often respond to flower essences far more strongly and easily than adults. And essence testing is less time consuming than MAP or MAP/Calibration sessions. So, first try several essence dosages.

If you have questions about whether a specific problem should be addressed with essences or with MAP or MAP/Calibration, you can open a MAP coning with your child's team (without the child being present) and ask the questions. It is essentially like a consultation call.

If you wish to incorporate MAP in your child's health care program, do the scanning session and several regular sessions with the child as soon as possible to get the team set up and to get you comfortable with working with the team. Don't wait for the child to get sick before doing this.

ADMINISTERING FLOWER ESSENCES TO CHILDREN: In general, a child up to the age of nine months can receive flower essences either orally *or* on the forehead. Their nervous system is still quite sensitive and can easily receive essences through the skin on the forehead area.

For a child older than nine months, it is best to give the essences orally. You can cut the alcohol- or vinegar-preservative taste by diluting the solution in a little bit of water—about a quarter of a cup. But the child will need to take all of this solution. You can also dilute the solution in water or juice in their bottle. They don't need to guzzle it all at once.

In a MAP session: For children from birth to four years old who are asleep, the essences can be administered on the forehead. The teams are able to assist the absorption of the essences into the electrical system for a child up to age four. Over age four, it is better to give the essence solution to them orally after they wake up the next morning.

Oh yes, here's one more piece of information about MAP teams for children. Several of the teams have included a big, overly lovable, huggable dog. It seems to be the same dog who works with a number of the children's teams. But she's been so helpful, I wouldn't be surprised if a MAP team canine corps has been established. Now, she doesn't function in a medical capacity (just in case you were wondering) but the teams have found that her presence is calming to some children. Often, children see her or feel her hot breath panting over them. Sometimes, even the parents have seen her or felt that breath. And they've said that their child visibly relaxes when she is around. So, if your child talks about a dog on the team, that's not his imagination running rampant!

SURROGATING MAP FOR ADULTS

Let's get real here. MAP is a very simple process. If a person is too ill or injured to activate and participate in sessions on their own, and they would like MAP's help, you can help them by using the Emergency MAP Procedure. Other than this, there's really no need to surrogate MAP for an adult. It is very important that an adult interested in MAP really wants it enough to initiate it. This program has to hit a person in their heart, soul, and gut. If someone who is perfectly capable of following the simple MAP steps is asking you to surrogate them for you, it is probably a sign that they really don't want to be in the program. They are hesitating and they need more time. The MAP steps could not be easier, but the program itself takes time, effort, intent, and diligence on the person's part. They need to be wholeheartedly committed. Encourage them to back off, and let them know that backing off is really okay.

The best way to help someone get into MAP is to spend time going over the steps with them. Tell them how easy it is to open a coning. Talk to them about your experiences in opening a coning. Show them kinesiology and work with them on it. Talk about flower essences. And talk about your MAP experiences. But don't just leave it at that. Either loan the person your copy of the *MAP* book or get another copy for them. Don't let them jump into the program with just your understanding of the steps and your experiences. Be sure they have the book with all the steps as they are to be followed and

179

the more complete information about the program itself
for reference.

Chapter 8

Quick Reference Steps

IMPORTANT: Do not do these steps without first reading this book. The information contained in the book is vital to your understanding of the process and the steps.

FIRST SESSION: THE SCANNING SESSION

(Do not use these steps before reading Chapter 3.)

1. Lie on your back with a blanket close at hand.

2. Open the coning. Wait 10 seconds after each connection. State:

> I'd like to open a MAP coning. I'd like to connect with:
> Overlighting Deva of Healing
> Pan
> White Brotherhood Medical Unit
> My higher self

Wait another 10–15 seconds.

3. During the scanning session, you do not need to talk. Remain still for one hour. At the end of the hour,

request that you be given a symbol or word or sensation to be used as identification for your team.

4. Close the coning. Spend a few minutes quietly.

Wait 24 hours before the second session.

REGULAR SESSIONS

(Do not use these steps before reading Chapters 3 and 4.)

Lie down or sit comfortably with a blanket and have the flower essences handy.

1. Open a MAP coning:
   Overlighting Deva of Healing
   Pan
   White Brotherhood Medical Team (Visualize or say
       your identification code.)
   Your higher self
Wait 10–15 seconds.

2. Test for essences. Take what is needed. Do not test for dosage.

3. Focus attention on the medical team and describe *fully* how you are feeling. Tell them everything that comes to mind. Give feedback on any sensations, pleasant or difficult, that you feel during the session. The session lasts 40 minutes.

4. At the end of 40 minutes, thank your team and end the session by closing the coning. Disconnect from each member of the coning individually.

5. Test yourself for flower essences and check for dosage. Spend a few minutes quietly.

MAP/CALIBRATION COMBINED SESSIONS

(Do not use these steps before reading Chapters 3, 4, and 5.)

Lie down or sit comfortably with a blanket and have the flower essences handy.

1. Open a MAP coning:
   Overlighting Deva of Healing
   Pan
   White Brotherhood Medical Team (Visualize/say
      your identification code.)
   Your higher self
   Wait 10–15 seconds.

2. Test for essences. Take what is needed. Do not test for dosage.

3. State:
   "I'd like to open to Pan for the Calibration Process.
      I'd like that special connection to occur now."
   Wait 5–10 seconds or use kinesiology to verify.

4. Explain to both your team and Pan what your difficulty is. Describe *fully* how you are feeling. Tell them

everything that comes to mind. Give feedback on any sensations you feel during the session. The combined session lasts 40 minutes.

5. To end the session, thank everyone and close down the coning by disconnecting from:

> Overlighting Deva of Healing
> Pan *from within the Calibration Process link*
> Pan *from within the MAP coning*
> Your White Brotherhood Medical Team
> Your higher self

6. Test yourself for essences and dosage. Spend a few minutes quietly.

EMERGENCY MAP PROCEDURE

(Do not use these steps before reading Chapters 3, 4, and 6.)

1. Open the coning by stating: "I want to open an Emergency MAP coning with the _____ team." (Insert code name of your team.)

2. Take one dropperful of ETS (Emergency Trauma Solution) every 3–5 minutes for the first 20 minutes after a trauma has occurred.

3. After the 20 minutes, and if able, test for essences for the specific trauma. Make a solution. Take this solution every 30–40 minutes for the next 2–3 hours.

4. Stay connected with the Emergency MAP coning and team throughout the time it takes you to stabilize from the emergency. This includes any hospitalization.

5. Once stabilized (or at home), get a follow-up MAP schedule and close the Emergency MAP coning. Test yourself for essences and dosage.

SURROGATING EMERGENCY MAP

(Do not use these steps before reading Chapters 3, 4, and 6.)

1. If possible, clear yourself with flower essences before beginning.

2. TO OPEN THE CONING FOR SOMEONE ALREADY IN MAP:

a) State: "I want to open an Emergency MAP coning with the _____ team." (Insert name of person's team or name of person, if you don't know the code.)

TO OPEN A CONING FOR SOMEONE WHO DOES NOT HAVE A MAP TEAM:

a) Get conscious permission to open an Emergency MAP coning.

b) Once permission is granted, open the coning. State: "I want to open an Emergency MAP coning for ____ ." (Insert name of person in trouble.)

3. Administer their ETS (Emergency Trauma Solution) to them, if possible. If there is no pre-mixed ETS and

you have your flower essences available, do a surrogate basic test and give the person any needed essences. Then telegraph test the essences *for their initial shock,* and administer this solution to them every 3–5 minutes for the first 20 minutes.

4. After the 20 minutes, telegraph test for essences for the specific trauma. Make a solution. Administer this solution every 30–40 minutes for the next 2–3 hours. Test yourself for flower essences periodically to ensure you are clear.

5. Once the person is stabilized (or at home), close the Emergency MAP coning. Test the person for essences and dosage. If he wishes to get into MAP on his own, give him the book and help him understand the steps.

NOTE: If you are unable to test for essences, just do steps 2 and 5, skipping steps 1, 3 and 4.

SURROGATING MAP FOR CHILDREN

(Do not use these steps before reading Chapters 3, 4, and 7.)

THE SCANNING SESSION

1. a) Open a children's MAP coning. (Wait 10 seconds after each connection.)
   Overlighting Deva of Healing
   Pan
   White Brotherhood Medical Unit

Your higher self

The child's higher self

Wait another 10–15 seconds.

b) Inform the White Brotherhood that you are acting on behalf of this child.

c) Test yourself for essences and take what is needed. Do not test for dosage. The child does not have to be tested at this point for the scanning session.

2. Scan the child with both hands.

3. Session lasts one hour. At the end, ask for the child's team code.

4. Close the coning.

5. Test yourself for essences and check for dosage. Then test the child for essences and dosage.

REGULAR CHILDREN'S MAP SESSION

1. a) Have the flower essences handy. Open the children's MAP coning using the child's team code, if you have it.

Overlighting Deva of Healing

Pan

White Brotherhood Medical Team

(Visualize team code.)

Your higher self

The child's higher self

Wait 10–15 seconds.

b) Test yourself for essences and take what is needed. Then, if essences can be administered, test the child for essences and give what is needed. Do not test for dosage for you or the child.

2. Regular sessions last 40 minutes. Tell the team the state of the child's health. Be prepared to assist and offer support. Take notes. Ask questions. Get any prescribed treatments or changes.

3. Close down the coning. Check both yourself and the child for essences and dosages.

SURROGATING MAP FOR ADULTS

1. Don't. In an emergency, follow the Surrogating Emergency MAP steps. (See page 185.)

Chapter 9

Professional
MAP Teams

We are presently involved in the transition from the Piscean to the Aquarian era. This shift requires us to develop a new intellectual outlook and new ways of working with and within the Aquarian dynamic. *Everything* is moving through this transition. This includes our physical body. Even on a cellular level we are now responding to the new, and moving away from the old.

This change has created an ever-widening gap in our health care systems. To be effective during the Piscean era, our allopathic and alternative modalities had to address healing balance within the Piscean dynamic. What we have now are allopathic and alternative health systems that address balance from the Piscean perspective. At the same time, we have a growing number of people who are altering the balance and rhythm of their bodies and lifestyles in response to the Aquarian dynamic. This has created a gap in health care. Systems and modalities that worked well even ten years ago are less effective today. Some health care practitioners recognize this and are trying mightily to address it. But for the most part, they are operating on a wing and a prayer and with good intentions—hoping what they are doing differently will be helpful.

All health care practices must now correspond to the Aquarian transition dynamic. Old definitions, approaches, and expectations must be replaced with new ways of thinking and doing.

Working with a Professional MAP team is the most effective way to make these changes because the White Brotherhood Medical Unit and nature fully understand the new era we are moving into and what changes we have to make during the transition. They have the knowledge, understanding, and ability to create structures that support us through the transition. And— equally important—they are eager to work with us in a professional capacity to do just this if we consciously request their assistance.

If you are a health care practitioner and want to include the new Aquarian health and healing dynamics in your practice, you may work with a Professional MAP team. This team is different from your personal MAP team because its focus will be the direction and nature of your professional work.

Here's what you do:

1. You must establish a *personal* MAP team and move through the initial five-month program outlined in this book. Besides stabilizing and balancing your health,

this will give you ample time to learn to work with MAP.

2. After the five months, if you would like to work with a Professional MAP team but you are not yet confident or comfortable working with your personal team, take more time to gain this confidence and comfort. Take all the time you need. The critical issue is the development of your ability to communicate effectively with your team and your physical ability to function within a coning for a specific period of time. You will not be able to work with a Professional MAP team unless you can communicate with them (using kinesiology is fine) and work in the coning for long periods of time. So, the time you spend developing your ability to stabilize physically while in a coning and developing the different skills in your working relationship with your personal team builds the foundation you need to work with the professional team.

Once you are comfortable working with your personal team, open the following MAP coning (you are *not* connected to your personal MAP team when doing this):

Overlighting Deva of Healing

Pan

White Brotherhood Medical Unit

Your higher self

If this sounds familiar it is because this is how you opened the first coning for the scanning session with MAP.

3. Tell this group that you want to work with a Professional MAP team to shift your practice to the new medical dynamics. Then describe the area of health care you work in. By the time you have finished defining or describing your work, you will be connected to your Professional MAP team. It will be comprised of members of the White Brotherhood Medical Unit who work specifically in your area.

4. Request a professional team code. You will now have two codes. One you will use when connecting with your personal team, and the other you will use when connecting with your professional team. When you work with a professional team, you do not drop your personal team. The professional team works solely with you in the development and implementation of the new dynamics in your health care practice. It also works with you as the practitioner. Your personal team will continue to work with you for illnesses, imbalances, personal emotional processes, and other areas of personal growth. In short, you will continue addressing the same kinds of issues with your personal team as you did prior to opening a professional team.

5. Begin to get acquainted. Ask questions you have regarding working together. Ask if they have suggestions for you about setting up this working relationship. Use this session to lay as much of the groundwork for working together as you can. Ask about how often you should meet and time limits for the working sessions. NOTE: They may want to wait until after the monitoring

session (explained in the next paragraph) to work out the meeting schedule with you. Just ask the team if they would like to wait before discussing a session schedule. If you communicate through kinesiology, word your questions in the simple yes/no format.

THE MONITORING SESSION: They will want to monitor you at work before giving you any work-related suggestions, and possibly prior to setting up a meeting schedule, so plan a time with them when they can do this monitoring session.

For the monitoring, all you need to do is open your Professional MAP team coning (using their code name) prior to seeing a client. (You do not need to do this in front of the client. The team will be monitoring your work and how the client responds. It will not be working personally with the client. Therefore, no permission is needed from the client.) The team will take it from there. After the client leaves, you can either close the coning, leave it open for a second client monitoring (if you have one coming in right away), or have a question-and-answer session with your team about any changes they might suggest in your approach based on what they have already seen. If they were only able to monitor your work with one client, ask your team if they would like to monitor additional clients. If they do, ask how many more clients the team would like to monitor, and have those sessions as soon as possible. (If using kinesiology, you get this information by doing sequential testing. This is explained in Appendix C, Testing for Dosage.)

6. When working with the professional team during regular office sessions, you will open the coning at the beginning of your workday. You must remember to close the coning at the end of each day when you are finished working—*do not leave it open all night.* An open coning such as this will unnecessarily drain your energy. You will feel dog tired.

Pay attention to your energy level when you first begin to work with your Professional MAP team. You may be able to keep the coning open easily for half your day or a quarter of your day. But if you try to keep the coning open for the entire day, you might feel drained. This is because your "muscles" are not yet fully conditioned. So, work with the coning in the beginning only as long as you are physically capable. If you are not clear about the state of your "conditioning," ask your professional team how long they suggest you work in an activated coning in the beginning. In time, your conditioning will automatically strengthen, and you'll easily be able to keep the coning open for the full workday.

NOTE: Check yourself for flower essences every day just after opening and closing this coning. Flower essences will help balance you while you work in the coning. And, if after a while you feel your conditioning is not strengthening, ask your team what you need to do to assist this process. You may need a diet change or more sleep—something simple such as this.

IMPORTANT: The MAP teams do not want your client's higher self in the coning while he is being worked on, *unless he has given his conscious consent* to be included in the coning. As I have already stated, the MAP team is working with the practitioner and is not the client's personal team. To obtain conscious consent you have to explain to your client that you are working in a new manner and with a different kind of team, and give him a general idea of what is involved with a coning. You do not have to explain MAP since the team will not be working directly with the client. Once he has a basic understanding, he can decide whether he wants his higher self in the coning. *IMPORTANT: When the appointment is over, and before your client leaves your office, you must disconnect his higher self from the coning. Do not work with another client with someone else's higher self in the coning.*

To include a client's higher self in the MAP coning, just ask that the person's higher self be included in the already opened coning. This will occur immediately. To disconnect that higher self, simply ask that it disconnect from the coning. The coning can be modified in this manner, without having to create and dismantle it, every time you include someone's higher self. In other words, you do not have to open a coning from scratch or close the whole thing down if all you want to do is either add or subtract a client's higher self from that coning.

It would be good to test your client for flower essences just after including him in the coning and again after disconnecting him from the coning. A dosage should be tested for on the last test. This way you can ensure the client is fully stabilized during and after the coning experience.

The Professional MAP teams recommend that when you expand your practice to include them you inform your clients that you are changing how you work. Let them know that they may observe differences and that they should give you as much feedback as possible about differences they perceive in themselves. It would be helpful to assure your clients that you are available to them if they need to call. Some of their reactions to the new work may be dramatic and unexpected, and additional support from you would be appreciated. In short, let them know you are moving into something new and that you want them to feel comfortable with it and participate as much as possible.

Opening a Professional MAP team is easy. What is challenging is establishing a good, effective, working team that includes you. One thing you will feel right away is your team's eagerness to work with you professionally and support you as you go through the changes needed to work with them. To create an effective team, you must understand that *you* are a partner. Your team will be working with you in two ways:

1. while you work with clients;

2. during private meetings with your team to work out changes and new approaches, discuss the physical setup and possible changes needed in your office space, and discuss issues with specific clients. This team works with you professionally and not on you personally.

Get into a rhythm with your team. Open the coning whenever you are with a client, and then meet with your team regularly for additional input, change, and insight. You can ask your team how often you should meet with them.

NOTE: Sometimes you may ask your team for insight or understanding about a new procedure or result, and feel that they really don't want to answer your questions. If you "hear" your team, you can literally hear them back off from the questions. This is because you need to *observe* what's going on for a while before you can understand the answer to the questions. When we work in new areas, we sometimes don't understand what is going on because our understanding is based on logic built around old ways of doing things. So, if you sense them saying "Not yet," take the hint. You may need to observe something for a week, a month, even a year before you are able to understand answers to your questions.

The following is not a suggestion; it is a requirement. Keep good notes. Keep notes about changes in your work, responses and reactions of clients, and information you get from your team during meetings. The biggest surprise shared by nearly every practitioner who is working with a Professional MAP team is the massive amount of information and insights they (the practitioner) are suddenly faced with. This is like entering medical school. And not only will you need to keep good notes, you will have to organize them. Either keep them on computer or in a loose-leaf notebook to allow you to separate and shift blocks of notes around. You will want to refer back to these notes. Although this sounds tedious and time consuming, trying to find a specific piece of information from a 400-page stack of scribbled notes that have no sense of organization about them is a horror show. Believe it or not, the record-and-notes issue is the thing that most often breaks the back of the aspiring Professional MAP team participant. So, right from the beginning, spend time thinking about how you want to set up this note-keeping business. Make it easy, convenient and superorganized. Then once you figure out what you'd like, buy the stuff you need and use it. HINT: If you are using your carefully planned record-keeping system and find it isn't quite working the way you had hoped it would, quickly modify what you've set up. The Professional MAP program isn't something that lasts for a week or a month. It is a long-term program. So keep working on this until you find the record-keeping system that is comfortable for you.

Other points: Good notes organize your experience internally and externally. A lot will be happening and it will be helpful to keep a chronology of the changes, reactions, and information. You will also want to refer to your notes when you realize your perception wasn't accurate. Knowing how you perceived what the team said will help correct the error and understand how you got it wrong. That way you learn from mistakes and continue fine-tuning your working relationship with your team.

It is easy to work with your team around such issues as how to change existing procedures if you organize your information. For example, let's say the team wants you to alter your basic office procedure. You got this by asking about the office procedure in yes/no questions and using kinesiology. Suddenly you are faced with a large block of information—your entire office procedure—and you haven't a clue about how to change it. Get pencil and paper, then list your office procedure step by step, starting from the moment the person walks in the door. Number each individual step and don't include two steps together. Then, with your team, go down the list, read each step, and ask if that step is to be changed. If you get a yes, check the step. You'll most likely find your entire procedure does not have to be changed, but just a few steps. Focus on each step needing change and ask the team to give you insight about the change. Tell them what comes to mind and then test to see if your perception is accurate. Work with them on each step until you verify that you fully understand the changes. Then move on to the next step. When you have finished, read your new procedure step by step, testing each step as you go along. ("Is this step now complete?") If you get a negative response, this means that step needs to be further modified. Keep doing this until all the steps test positive.

One of the important keys to working with your team is good information management, and modifying your office procedure is a good example of this. Whenever you are dealing with a large comprehensive block of information, just break it down into simple, manageable pieces and work with one small piece at a time.

Start working with your team in a way that you feel is comfortable and reasonable. Don't feel you have to change how you work with all your clients right away. Do it in manageable increments and with clients with whom you feel most comfortable about making changes.

TIPS ABOUT WORKING IN A CONING

You don't want to remain in a coning longer than necessary. If you have one client scheduled in the morning and three clients scheduled in late afternoon, open the coning for the early client and then close the coning until the start of the afternoon sessions.

For days when clients are scheduled back to back, open the coning for the first client and leave it open throughout the day until the last client leaves. Then close the coning. It takes more effort and energy to open a coning than to sustain it. So you don't want to keep opening and closing conings throughout a day. However, you also don't want to expend energy to sustain the coning for unnecessarily long periods of time. You're going to have to use your judgment here. Your Professional MAP team can help you reach a balance if you are having trouble.

If you have the coning open all day, you don't need to keep it "active" during lunch. You can put a coning in an "at-rest" position simply by letting your team know you're going to lunch now (or whatever) and you'd like them to move into the at-rest position. You will feel an immediate easing within you. This way, you leave the coning open while expending very little energy to sustain it. After lunch, when you are getting ready for the next client, just tell the coning you're ready to work again, and you'll feel an activation as they respond.

You can ask your team any question at any time while the coning is open and fully activated—that is, not in an "at-rest" position. You don't have to do any kind of preparation to talk with them. Once the coning is open, they are with you at all times

Working in a coning for long periods of time may cause a protein drain. Be aware of how you feel, and increase your protein intake on the days you are working with your Professional MAP team.

WHAT TO EXPECT WHEN WORKING WITH A PROFESSIONAL MAP TEAM

1. Expect very different results than you are used to. For example, herbologists using kinesiology will get different results that will make little, if any, sense regarding which herbs to use. If you are working in a system that has an established tradition of how elements such as herbs are used and what they work with, you have to

disregard this information and allow new information to form.

2. Expect different, sometimes unusual, and sometimes strong responses and reactions to your work. MAP works in a more profound and comprehensive manner than you are used to. You may have deeper and different responses than clients formerly had. And the results can come more quickly than you are used to. You'll probably notice that your clients are more responsive to the new work.

Because of this, it is important that you offer support to your clients beyond the office. *You* may be surprised at what you see happening, but your client might be frightened at the suddenness and intensity.

3. You will get strong intuitive "hits" regarding what you are doing with a client. Learn to go with these hits. This is one way your team works with you. If you are questioning the hit, verify it with your team prior to doing anything. Quietly ask if what you are perceiving is correct, then describe what you are perceiving and either listen for their answer or test using kinesiology.

Expect the session to move differently. You will feel your team help as you move along. Be prepared to change how you function in a session. You may receive a strong urging to do something you would not normally consider. In these cases, trust your intuition and just do it. The proof of its accuracy will be in the results.

4. Give the team complete descriptions of your patient's condition. Don't just say, "Sam has glaucoma." "Piscean glaucoma" is different and manifests differently than "Aquarian glaucoma." So when talking about a specific condition with your team, give detailed descriptions of the symptoms.

5. Expect a change in clientele. We are in a transition time. People who need a Piscean modality may no longer be comfortable with you and may seek another practitioner. Understand that this might happen and give them a graceful way out. It would be helpful if you put together, for these clients, a list of practitioners who you feel work in the Piscean framework and whom you recommend.

NOTE. Those who have begun working with teams report that there *is* a shift in clients but that they end up drawing far more new clients to them. I think there are more people than we realize out there who need this new work and will immediately be drawn to it once they know it is available.

6. Expect personal changes as you create and develop this teamwork and the new health system moves along. Use flower essences to help stabilize yourself and remember to bring any personal issues to your *personal* MAP team. You won't be eliminating your personal team when you begin working with the professional team. In fact, you may work with your personal team even more. If you are frightened and resistant, and throwing up blocks around the changes that are being

suggested in your practice, you can do a MAP/Calibration with your personal team. You will have personal responses to the inevitable growing pains and discomfort at working in the dark.

7. Expect resistance on your part. If you spent years diligently learning a health care system, you will, from time to time, dig your heels in and resist changes your team suggests. This is especially true when the practitioner who opens to the new team has established a reputation. Fear comes up about the possibility of losing recognition or tarnishing a reputation. Also, for a person to work with the MAP team, he has to release a lot of previous knowledge. This, too, can result in a lot of heel digging.

As mentioned above, one excellent way to deal with resistance is to do a MAP/Calibration with your personal team. Do this as soon as you recognize resistance.

8. Do not work in a professional team coning while simultaneously having a personal team coning open. Open and work with one coning or the other, not both.

9. The impressions shared with me about Professional MAP teams indicates that they are excited and anxious to work with us—and they are funny! A number of people have talked about their terrific humor. They are also polite, considerate, and caring. However, they will push you a little to keep you moving with the changes.

Perhaps the best thing I've heard many say about Professional MAP is that it is not for the fainthearted.

It's amazing to me how often I hear this. People usually get into Professional MAP with the expectation that it will be easy—and immediately are struck by a very different experience. Professional MAP is exciting, exhilarating, demanding, incredibly educational, often amazing, tedious, frustrating, time consuming, and sometimes scary. One thing that I think everyone experiencing it would agree on is that it is not easy. The teams are helping you to restructure your health discipline. You will be receiving a huge amount of information, and you will need to test it, work with it, and then integrate it into your practice. There will be times when you will have received so much information that you will need to put the whole thing away and take a breather. This is an *intense* partnership. But many who have stayed with it talk about how liberating this partnership is. You no longer have to know it all. Now you will be working with a team that has the information. You don't have to research beyond this. You couldn't have a better professional partner than a Professional MAP team.

QUICK REFERENCE STEPS FOR OPENING
A PROFESSIONAL MAP TEAM CONNECTION

(Do not use these steps until after reading this chapter.)

1. Establish a personal MAP team and move through the initial five-month program outlined in this book. Before moving on to Professional MAP, make sure you have a comfortable and confident relationship with your personal MAP team.

2. Open the following MAP coning:
   Overlighting Deva of Healing
   Pan
   White Brotherhood Medical Unit
   Your higher self
   Wait 10–15 seconds. Then, test yourself for essences.

3. State that you want to work with a Professional MAP team to shift your practice to the new medical dynamics. Describe the health care area you work in.

4. Request a professional team code.

5. Get acquainted. Ask pertinent questions regarding your schedule for setting up Professional MAP team meetings. Schedule one or more monitoring sessions when you will be working with clients.

6. Thank your new team. Close the coning as you would a personal MAP coning. Test yourself for flower essences and dosage.

FOR REGULAR PROFESSIONAL MAP TEAM SESSIONS: Open a Professional MAP coning using your professional team code name. Test yourself for essences. If you are seeing clients, go about your day, but be aware of any assistance your team might be offering. After the last client, close down the coning. Test for essences and dosage if you are not planning to be in the office for a few days. If you are scheduled to be in the office the next day, you do not need to test for dosage. The next day's tests will pick up any needed essences.

For meetings in which you plan to work with your team outside client visits, simply open the team coning. Test for flower essences. Have your discussion and meeting for however long you wish. Then close the coning and test essences again. Check for dosage if you don't plan to have a professional session the next day.

The following is a portion of a letter I received from an acupuncturist practicing in Ireland. She had been working diligently with her Professional MAP team for about six months when she wrote this. I felt her experiences might be helpful to others.

Here I'll interject something that may be useful to others—namely, how I ask clients in this conservative area if I can connect to their higher self. After I've done my normal diagnostic work, involving lots of questions and a physical exam, I tell the client that my intent, in all my work, is to work in harmony with that highest part of themselves, however they conceive of it—their spirit, their soul, their higher self. I say that I feel I can do this most effectively if I inwardly ask to consciously connect with them at that level whenever they are here for a treatment. I ask them if that is alright. When I use this approach, there is unanimous consent—usually with genuine appreciation. I then inwardly do the connecting and disconnecting at each session. This approach has the okay of my Professional MAP team.

There are a few clients who I do inform of my work with nature and MAP. Mostly, however, I don't. I think that over time there will be more and more clients I can share with more openly. Naturally, in these cases, I encourage them to work with MAP and essences so as to be able to work on their own as much as they choose and not be dependent on me.

Other specific techniques I'm working on with my Professional MAP team include having more than one coning at once. (I have two treatment rooms and sometimes have two clients at the same time—but I don't want the higher self of one to be involved with the other.) I explained to my team what I need, and I have their okay to set up a coning and identify it according to the higher self of the client with whom I'm working. (I just open the initial four-point Professional MAP coning once at the start of the day, and add the client's higher self. Then, if I'm using the second room, I tell my team I need a second treatment room coning *without* John's higher self, and *with* Mary's higher self. If I'm in the room with Mary, and need to get information regarding John (e.g., "Are John's needles ready to come out now?"), I'll ask to switch to John's treatment room coning and then kinesiology test for whatever information I need.

Professional MAP teams are not for the fainthearted. It's very difficult to know what's going on when a patient *doesn't* do well after a treatment. Worst of all, it's hard to rely on my kinesiology testing when I'm asking questions like, "Did I make a mistake in my kinesiology testing for John's treatment?" Usually, I find this is a person I am not supposed to treat. I now try to remember to test for this question before I schedule someone's first appointment. That way, I can refer them to another health professional.

C. O., Ireland

A NOTE ABOUT PROFESSIONAL MAP: We have established a Professional MAP networking list. If you would like to be on the list and have your contact information made available to other Professional MAP practitioners, just drop us a note letting us know. (This information will not be given to those just working with a personal MAP team.) We suggest that you also let us know what professional discipline you are working in with your team.

If you would like information about other Professional MAP practitioners in your geographic area, let us know this also. We do not automatically send this information when you request to be put on the list.

The Professional MAP networking list is offered so professionals can share with other professionals how they have used MAP in their practices. We ask those requesting it to use it for professional networking only, and not for any advertising or marketing purposes. However, we cannot *guarantee* that everyone will honor this request.

A FINAL NOTE: The Professional MAP procedure described in this chapter is the same procedure used for working with a nature/White Brotherhood team in non-medical professions. In these cases, you set up a coning that specifically applies to the profession you are interested in. (You do *not* set up a Professional MAP coning for a non-medical profession.) For instructions on how to set up a non-medical professional coning, see Appendix A.

Chapter 10

Sharing MAP
with Others

If you wish to share MAP with others, it is *vital* that you make this entire book available to them and not just the quick-reference MAP steps or your verbal rendition of the steps. It is important that anyone using MAP has the information contained in the book as a foundation. Everyone who gets into the program needs to be fully informed. And they need the information to be unfiltered. This is so they can develop their own relationship with their team in a balanced and safe MAP environment. To give someone just the steps would place them at a serious disadvantage, lead to possible misinterpretation of the steps, and possibly cause them difficulties. MAP is a potent tool and should not be entered lightly nor should it be shared with others in a haphazard manner.

MAP may be the best thing to come along for you. Your life may change in dramatic and exciting ways once you start the work. Because of this, you may have a burning desire to share MAP with everyone you know—and maybe even some you don't know. I ask you to be sensitive about sharing MAP. If you don't know for sure that the other person would be comfortable with the MAP concept and its information, think about it before talking to the person. If you know from past experience that this person will challenge and resist what you would like to say, back off. MAP is a program that is to be embraced heart and soul. It is not a program to sell, convince, or do battle over.

INTRODUCING MAP TO A FRIEND: Besides giving or loaning the friend the book (or suggesting they buy their own copy), you can help by sharing your MAP experiences with this person. Also, if you are using kinesiology and flower essences, it would be especially good to demonstrate both of these things and help them through their learning process.

INTRODUCING MAP TO AN INFORMAL GROUP: If you wish to present MAP to a group of acquaintances and friends, we ask that you make the book available to the participants at the time of the presentation. Again, it is important that people have access to the full information about MAP and not have to depend on another person's personal interpretation of the program. Sharing the book, your personal experiences, and demonstrating kinesiology and how to test for flower essences would give them an excellent start to the program. It would also be best if you, as the presenter, have at least six-months experience with your MAP team before presenting MAP in an informal group context. Please contact us at Perelandra for details on making the book available to groups.

GIVING A MAP WORKSHOP: I don't feel a person is qualified to give a MAP workshop unless they have been working diligently in the program for at least two years. When a person offers a workshop, he implies a certain expertise. I happen to know that there are a number of people who do not meet this criteria and, because they are excited about "spreading the word" or wish to make an easy buck off MAP, feel the need to start a little cottage industry around giving MAP workshops. So, if you think you might like to give a MAP or MAP-related workshop, please meet this two-year-minimum criteria.

The second criteria is that the *MAP* book be made available at the workshop and the participants who are interested in getting into MAP are encouraged to buy the book. (Contact Perelandra for information about purchasing in quantity.)

The following is an outline for MAP workshops given by two people that is both well put together and maintains the integrity of MAP. If you are inclined to offer the program as a workshop, I suggest this format and setup. It has proven to be clear and helpful.

1. Step-by-step overview of the MAP program. In this part each step is given *as written* and discussed. Also include discussions about the White Brotherhood, nature, why both of these groups are involved in a medical program, coning, involution/evolution balance, and how the White Brotherhood and nature create involution/evolution balance in the MAP coning.

2. Tips on working with your MAP team. The areas of discussion are taken from Chapter 4 and discussed according to what is written in that chapter and the presenter's personal experiences. Also make sure the participants understand that MAP can be used in conjunction with a doctor's care and how to weave the program in with other trained health care professionals when needed. Make sure they do not feel they must choose one over the other.

3. Using kinesiology to communicate with your MAP team and test flower essences. This includes a demonstration of kinesiology and a discussion of the technique and problems they might have with the technique. The information for this and how to test the essences is in Appendices B and C, and expanded on by the presenter's personal experiences with kinesiology and flower essences. Helping people in a group context to learn kinesiology is easy—after all, it is an easy tool. And it's especially helpful to others because, for some reason, people who do not hesitate for a second to get into MAP will hesitate greatly to learn kinesiology on their own.

4. Fundamentals of flower essences and how they are used in MAP. The basis for this discussion is in Appendix B and also draws from your personal experiences. The book *Flower Essences* is also helpful.

5. Optional: the Emergency MAP Procedure and how to test for the ETS. A presentation and discussion of the steps and a demonstration of how to test for and make the ETS can be helpful.

Now, just because I am suggesting a workshop outline does not mean that I want a bunch of people running around giving MAP workshops. On the contrary, I think the book is self-explanatory. But, I've been somewhat dismayed at what some people are doing to MAP, and I've come to realize that it is inevitable that people are going to want to present the program. I thought if you knew what criteria I feel are important for the presenter and the information that I think should be presented, perhaps we'd have better quality and more responsible activity in this area.

IMPORTANT: Do not open a MAP coning for a group. First of all, this is a misuse of the MAP coning and the teams. MAP is not a group experience. It is a medical program for individuals. Secondly, there are too many unknown variables in a group such as this to assure a safe environment for opening something as powerful as a MAP coning. Someone could panic and experience difficulty. The MAP coning and its members can be discussed in a group context, but the coning itself should not be opened. (In Chapter 5, we talked about the Group Calibration Process, but that is not the same as using a MAP coning. See Chapter 5 if you need clarification on this. See also Appendix A on Conings.)

Lastly, *please* do not improvise or customize MAP. The MAP program is designed and developed by the White Brotherhood and nature team as it is presented in this book. This is how they wish the program to be used. It is constructed with a strong involution/evolution balance, which is the key to the program's success and ensures optimal safety, efficiency, and results. Tinkering with it to suit your personal desires can screw up this balance. If you are presenting the program to others, don't change the MAP steps, the language, or rename any of the team participants. If you are inclined to do these things, you are misrepresenting the program and can cause problems for others.

Chapter 11

Nature Healing Coning for Animals

MAP has been conceived and designed for human beings. It is not designed for nor can it accommodate animals. Just as a person would not take an injured or sick pet to a human's hospital emergency room, he should not take a pet to MAP. To put it simply: it is inappropriate. This is not to say that MAP is "too good" for animals. We are talking about two separate things here—animals and humans.

Since MAP was introduced to the public in 1990, a number of people have attempted to include their pets in the MAP program. Basically, what the MAP team does when presented with an animal is immediately "transfer the call" to the appropriate "department"—that is, nature.

When it comes to the health issues of animals, nature is the best and most efficient healing assistant. The MAP teams would not work with an animal if something or someone else would do a better job. And MAP *knows* nature is the best healing assistant for nature. (Remember, no matter how intelligent an animal is, it is an animal and not a furred or feathered human. Animals require different healing approaches. This is why vets go to veterinary schools to train and not to medical schools.)

You can set up a healing coning for an animal without involving MAP. In fact, it is more appropriate and efficient if the healing coning is set up by you directly and not set up in a second-hand way through MAP. There are two animal healing conings to choose from, and your choice will depend on whether or not you should participate in the healing session. In each procedure, I have included the option of flower essences testing.

FOR COMPANION ANIMALS

Use this coning when you know the animal, and you choose to participate in the healing process. Your participation is similar to how one participates in a MAP session for children. You will need to ask questions, and you may be asked to take the animal to the vet, if necessary, or give medicine or special food. Consulting nature will not interfere with consulting a vet. Use the Nature Healing Coning as part of the animal's regular health regime, in emergency situations, and during office visits. Set up the coning with the animal prior to surgery and hospital stays, then close the coning down after the animal is fully stabilized and after you have gotten the suggested schedule for additional nature coning sessions. Additional conings may be used throughout the healing process if needed. Also, the Nature Healing

Coning may be opened for the animal to assist it through death. Once the process is complete, simply close the coning—and test yourself for essences. (Also, see Chapter 8 in *Flower Essences* for assisting an animal through its death process.)

Nature Healing Coning for Companion Animals

1. Open a Nature Healing Coning. Wait 10 seconds after each connection is made.
   a) the Deva of Animal Healing
   b) Pan and/or the nature spirits working with this animal
   c) the higher self of the animal State: I want to be connected to _____'s higher self.
   d) your higher self

Allow another 10–15 seconds for the coning to fully activate and settle in. Test yourself for essences. You don't have to test the animal at this point.

2. Explain what you know and have observed about the animal's condition. Do this as fully as you can. Then sit quietly and let the coning work with the animal for 30 minutes. (Your explanation lets those in the coning know what you understand about the animal's condition. This is important since you will be participating in the animal's healing process.)

During this time, you may feel/sense/hear that you are to test the animal for flower essences. Ask the coning if your intuition is correct. Test using kinesiology. Give the animal a basic flower essence test and administer the essences that are needed. (Use the same surrogate testing process you would use for a human. See Appendix C.) Don't test for dosage at this point.

NOTE: The easiest way to administer essences to an animal is to make a small solution in about one-eighth of a cup of water, and squirt two or three dropperfuls of this solution into the animal's mouth using a clean *plastic* dropper.

3. At the end of the 30 minutes, ask the coning any questions that come to mind having to do with what the animal needs and how you may assist. Should the animal go to the vet? If so, should another Nature Healing Coning session be held after the vet visit? (Assume that the coning should be open during the vet visit.) Should the animal's diet be changed, and how? Is this change temporary? If so, how long should it go on? Should there be additional nature healing sessions even if the animal doesn't go to the vet? If so, how many and when? Continue asking questions until you feel you have all the information you need. (You can receive your information by asking questions in a simple yes/no format and testing with kinesiology.)

4. Test the animal for flower essences once more. Include a dosage test.

5. The session is now finished. It is important to disconnect or dismantle the Nature Healing Coning. Do this by asking each participant to disconnect, one by one

(the Deva of Animal Healing, Pan and/or the nature spirits working with this animal, the animal's higher self, and your higher self), from the coning. The session is over. Test yourself for flower essences and dosage.

FOR WILD ANIMALS

This coning is for those who wish to assist injured or sick wild animals, or other animals in need to whom you are a stranger and in whose healing process you will not be able to participate. In these cases, the only thing you have to offer is a healing coning. Most of the time, it is either impossible or not appropriate to follow up with any assistance on your part—such as giving medicine or taking the animal to the vet. Consequently, you (your higher self) do not have to be part of the coning. You won't be asking questions or receiving information. Although you need to be physically present when opening this coning, you do not have to be dangerously close to the animal. Use your common sense. Also, try to be present without alarming the animal. (If you *are* going to assist a wild animal through a healing process, use the Nature Healing Coning as set up for companion animals.) Here's what you do for wild animals:

1. Connect with the animal's higher self. (Do this exactly as you would when connecting to your pet's higher self—ask to be connected. Verify the connection using kinesiology.)

2. Ask if it is appropriate to assist this animal by opening a Nature Healing Coning.

If you get "no," go no further. The animal doesn't wish to be disturbed, doesn't want your assistance, and for you to proceed would be interference. Just disconnect from the animal's higher self and leave.

If you get "yes," go on to step 3.

3. Open a Nature Healing Coning. Do this by asking to be connected to:
   a) the Deva of Animal Healing
   b) Pan and/or the nature spirits working with this animal
   c) the higher self of the animal

Allow about 15 seconds for the coning to fully activate and settle in. (Your higher self is not included in this coning.)

4. The healing coning will know what to do for this animal. All you have to do is sit quietly for 30 minutes.

5. At the end of 30 minutes, you may wish to test the animal for flower essences. However, do not try to administer the essences in the mouth. Simply put the drops anywhere on the animal's body. With some wild animals, it may be dangerous or impossible to test and administer flower essences. If this is the case, skip this option.

6. Close the coning. Do this by asking each participant to disconnect, one by one (the Deva of Animal Healing, Pan and/or the nature spirits working with this

animal, and the animal's higher self), from the coning. The session is over.

7. Since you were not part of the coning, you don't need to test yourself for essences. However, if this experience was especially stressful for you, it would be a good idea to test them anyway.

NOTE: If you would like to learn more about using flower essences with animals, I recommend that you read the animal section in Chapter 8 in the book *Flower Essences*.

Appendices

Appendix A

Conings

The keystone of MAP is its coning. It is set up to assure perfect balance between the involution dynamic (nature) and the evolution dynamic (the White Brotherhood and you). The evolution dynamic supplies the purpose and definition to any thing or action. The involution dynamic (nature) supplies the matter, means, and action for achieving evolution's purpose and definition. The human soul is the force behind the evolution dynamic. Nature is the force behind involution. In health, the evolution dynamic comes from one's soul. It is from our soul that we receive the impulses that define our direction and our purpose. It is the soul that gives the necessary data to nature for all that is physically required for a human to fully operate within a given lifetime. Nature then supplies our body according to these soul-directed specifications. This also means that nature is the engineer of the human body, and like any good engineer, nature knows how it is supposed to work and how to fix it if it isn't working correctly.

Technically speaking, a coning is a balanced vortex of conscious energy. The simplest way to explain a coning is to say that it is a conference call. With a coning, we are working with more than one intelligence simultaneously.

The reason a coning is needed for multilevel processes is because of the greater stability, clarity, and balance it offers. With multilevel processes, we are working with many different facets and levels of intelligences at one time. Consequently, it is far better to work in an organized team comprised of all those involved in the area we are focusing on.

A coning, by nature, has a high degree of protection built into it. Because of the larger scope of the work, it is important to define exactly who and what are involved in that work. All others are excluded by the mere fact that they have not been activated in the coning. In essence, a coning creates not only the team but also the "room" in which the team is meeting. It is important, when activating a coning, to discern between those team members who are a part of the work to be done and those others who are not involved. The coning is created and activated by us—the human team member. Only those with whom we seek connection will be included. Members will not "slide" in and out of a coning on their own. This adds to the exceptional degree of protection contained within the coning.

I have said that a coning also offers balance and clarity. A friend of mine who began to use coning whenever she did multilevel work was quite impressed at the difference the coning made in both the quality of her work and the process she went through during her work. She said that when she began to do her work while in a coning, she felt as if she was sitting in a beautiful, sunlit room with the windows open and a lovely warm breeze softly blowing in. Before she learned to use a coning, she would just "connect in" with various "helpers." She said that, in comparison, it was as if she was sitting in a room with no windows and struggling to get a full breath of air. What she was describing was the contrast she felt with the balance and clarity the coning gave her.

Any combination of team members can be activated for the purpose of simultaneous input. But this does not constitute a coning. A true coning has balance built into it. By this I mean a balance between nature and the human soul. In order for us to experience anything fully, we must perceive it in a balanced state; that is, it must have an equal reflection of the soul or spirit dynamics (evolution) combined with an equal reflection of the form/nature dynamics (involution). I see this balance in the shape of a V.

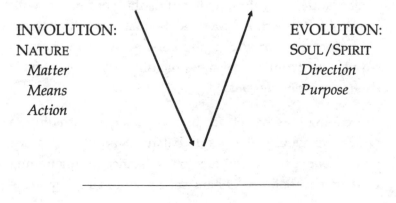

INVOLUTION:
NATURE
Matter
Means
Action

EVOLUTION:
SOUL/SPIRIT
Direction
Purpose

For anything to function well in form, it must have within it a balance between the involution dynamics and the evolution dynamics, or nature and spirit. The extent to which we achieve balance between the involution and evolution dynamics depends on our willingness to allow nature to be a partner with us. To have soul and spirit effectively, efficiently, and fully activated into form and action, one must have a balance between involution and evolution.

A coning is set up for the purpose of activating a team for specific work—in this case, MAP. It is therefore important for the successful completion of the work that a balance be maintained between the involution dynamics and the evolution dynamics within the coning itself. We do this by setting up a basic coning, which I call the "four-point coning," that lays a balanced foundation between the involution and evolution dynamics.

As a foundation, the four-point MAP coning maintains the necessary balance between (a) involution or nature, through the connection with the devic and nature spirit levels; and (b) evolution, through the connection with the White Brotherhood Medical Team and the higher self of the person working in the coning. We human souls supply the evolutionary dynamic only. *We cannot supply the involutionary dynamic.*

A coning may be set up for any project or situation in which we would like good, balanced input and assistance. People set up conings for assistance in functioning in their occupations. Others set up conings for starting

NATURE: INVOLUTION
1. *Devic Connection*
2. *Nature Spirit/Pan Connection*

SOUL/SPIRIT: EVOLUTION
3. *White Brotherhood*
4. *Our Higher Self*

and running their businesses. At Perelandra, we open a coning prior to all business meetings. With a coning, the meeting runs far more efficiently and decisions are more easily reached. The people who are participating in a coning work with the White Brotherhood to create and hold the appropriate vision and to define and give purpose to all that needs to be addressed. The people then work with nature to come up with solutions and courses of action that best supply the matter, means, action, and organization to what they wish to accomplish.

Anyone interested in functioning in harmony with the current transition from the Piscean dynamic to the Aquarian dynamic should include the White Brotherhood in any coning they activate. The White Brotherhood holds the major patterning and rhythms being utilized for this transition. They are part of a balanced coning because they support and assist in ensuring that any work conducted from the coning maintains its forward motion and its connection to the new Aquarian dynamic. For the purpose of a coning other than MAP, it is preferred that we ask, when opening a coning, to be

linked with the appropriate members of the White
Brotherhood working with _____ . (You define the
purpose and the area of focus of the coning.) The appropriate members will automatically be activated in the
coning. If you aren't clear about what or who to ask for,
just ask for a *general connection to the White Brotherhood.*
This will create a general, nonspecific connection with
them that will ensure that the evolutionary dynamic in
the coning is consistent with the intent and direction of
the new Aquarian shift.

In all conings, we include our higher self to assure
that the work done is compatible with *our* higher direction and purpose. This input is given automatically by
the fact that our higher self is linked into the coning.

The devic connection of the coning ensures that the
work being done maintains an overall integrity with
nature's design and direction in the area in which we are
working. The devic level also creates or designs appropriate courses of action and solutions to specific
situations or problems that need addressing. Each coning has in it a specific deva. For example, the MAP coning has the Overlighting Deva of Healing. (A deva is
"overlighting" if it is the "chief" deva of a larger devic
team. Each area of healing has its own deva. The deva
that "coordinates and oversees" all these areas is the
overlighting deva. But you don't have to get bogged
down with semantics. If you wish to work with the deva
of your business, or the deva of your home, or the deva
of the specific field of medicine you practice, just ask for
the deva of _____ . You don't have to know if it's over-

lighting or not. The deva knows this stuff.) When opening a coning, think about what issue or situation you
wish to address in the coning, then ask to be connected
with the deva of that specific issue or situation.

For some situations, you may need more than one
deva. A four-point coning only refers to the divisions of
the coning. It does not mean only four members can
participate in a coning. In some cases, you may need to
identify situations within larger contexts, and include
several devas as a result. For example, if I wish to work
in a coning with a specific vegetable in the Perelandra
garden, I will include the Deva of Perelandra, the Deva
of the Perelandra Garden, and the deva of the specific
vegetable in question. These three devas constitute one
point of the coning. And, the fact that I have three devas
"standing on that point," does not overload the point or
give it additional "weight." Another example: One of
my staff is putting together a co-creative staff team-
training program for us. To do this, she is working in a
coning. For the devic point, she has included the Deva
of Perelandra (this makes sure the overall direction of
Perelandra is maintained), the Deva of the Perelandra
Business (representing the business direction), and the
Deva of Team Development. These three devas combine
to create the appropriate team-development program for
the Perelandra business staff.

The nature spirit level of the coning is connected
through Pan. We do this because all nature spirits except
Pan are regional, and rather than try to figure out which
nature spirit or groups of nature spirits are involved in

the work we wish to do, we work with Pan—the one nature spirit who is universal in dynamic and is involved in all of the nature spirit activities. Because of this, we do not need to add additional nature spirits to this point. Pan's connection helps us maintain integrity with natural law for all action and issues worked on in the coning and gives assurance that the nature spirit activity and input is fully represented at all times.

STEPS FOR OPENING A FOUR-POINT CONING

Have your flower essences handy.

1. State: I wish to open a coning.

2. Link with each appropriate member of the coning individually:
   a) the specific deva(s) involved
   b) Pan
   c) the White Brotherhood—State: I'd like to be connected with the appropriate members of the White Brotherhood working with _____ .

For a non-medical professional White Brotherhood coning (as described in Chapter 9), state that you wish to shift your work to include the new Aquarian dynamic and want to work in a professional White Brotherhood team to accomplish this. Then describe your professional area.
   d) your higher self—State: I'd like my higher self to be connected to the coning.

Allow 10 seconds for each connection to occur. Then

verify that each connection has been made (using kinesiology) before going on to the next step. Wait another ten to fifteen seconds after activating the full coning so that your body can stabilize itself within the coning and with the team. (If you test that the coning is not activated, it is just because you were not focused during this step. Spend a moment collecting yourself, focus, and do this step again. Test again to verify.)

3. Test yourself for flower essences to make sure that the process of activating a coning did not affect your balance. Take any essences you tested positive for. You will not need to do a dosage test at this time for these essences because they are needed for one time only— while you are in the coning. To test yourself for essences, ask: Do I need any flower essences? (Test.)

If no, continue with the coning steps. If yes, test the essences.

4. Do the work or have the meeting you desire.

5. When the work is completed, thank your team for its assistance, and close down or dismantle the coning. *Closing down is important.* You do this simply by focusing on each member of the coning separately, thanking that member, and asking to be disconnected. Then verify that you are disconnected from each member by using kinesiology.

6. Test yourself for flower essences again, just to be sure that you held your balance once the coning work was completed. Take the essences that tested positive

235

and, this time, *check for dosage* to see if you will need to take the essence(s) more than one time.

If you have difficulty closing down the coning, and using kinesiology you keep getting a negative response to the question, "Am I disconnected from _____?", it is simply because you have temporarily lost your focus on what you are doing. No member of the coning is going to resist a disconnection any more than they would resist a connection. You are the one in command of the creation, activation, and dismantling of the coning. But you need to be connected to what you are doing. You can't let your mind drift. So, all you need to do when you are having a little trouble closing down is refocus yourself on what you are doing, request a disconnection again, and test to verify the disconnection. This time you will receive a positive verification.

Opening a Coning with More than One Person

The above steps are for opening a four-point coning when you are working by yourself. There will be times when you will need to work with more members and expand the team.

Also, there will be times when you will want to include other people in the coning. Once the four-point coning is open and activated, your stabilizing foundation is laid, and you may add any number of team members to that foundation. As already mentioned, the "four" in the four-point coning refers to the four levels of intelligences being activated: devic, nature spirit,

White Brotherhood, and you. You may have any number of participants within each of those levels. The four points as a unit will maintain their coning balance no matter how many participants are activated within the specific levels. So if you are working with a process that requires the deva of your business to be present, and two co-workers, Sally and Herbert, are present and participating with you during the process, you would:

1. Open the regular four-point coning: deva of the business, Pan, White Brotherhood, your higher self.

2. Ask that Sally's higher self be connected with the coning. Test to verify this connection. (This assumes you have Sally's *conscious* permission to include her higher self.)

3. Ask that Herbert's higher self be connected with the coning. Test to verify the connection. (This assumes you have Herbert's *conscious* permission to include his higher self.)

4. Test Sally, Herbert, and yourself for flower essences. Take the essences needed. Do not check for dosage.

5. You, Sally, and Herbert can now do the work or have the meeting.

6. Once the work is complete, thank the coning team, and dismantle the coning by asking to be disconnected from:
   Sally's higher self
   Herbert's higher self

Then, ask to disconnect the four-point coning:
  a) All devic connections, one at a time
  b) Pan/specific nature spirits
  c) White Brotherhood
  d) Your higher self

Test after each disconnection to make sure it has occurred.

7. Test Sally, Herbert, and yourself again for flower essences. Take those essences and check for dosage for each person to see if the essences need to be taken more than one time.

IMPORTANT POINTS ABOUT CONINGS

1. You may include as many members in your team as you like and maintain involution/evolution balance as long as you begin with the regular four-point coning as your foundation. However, it is best to include *only* those who are directly related to the work being done. Some people get a little crazy about coning activation and add forty-two members who might possibly be involved or might like to be involved. If you do, you no longer have a tight, cohesive team. You now have a mob coning instead.

I urge you to resist activating a mob coning for two reasons: a) It is totally unnecessary and does not strengthen or enhance a coning in any way. b) *You*, as the initiator and activator of the coning, will feel a substantial physical drain as you try to hold a coning with an unnecessary number of members present throughout the time it takes for the process or work. A coning, although invisible, is a physical energy reality that will interact with you. A mob coning would require the same amount of energy as trying to hold a deep conversation with six people in the middle of the New York Stock Exchange on Friday afternoon. You are going to feel exhausted from this kind of overload. So, the key to "good coning building" is to be precise about who you request to be on the team. Each member should have an integral role in the work to be done.

There's another point. *No person's higher self should be added into a coning without his or her conscious permission.* To do so without conscious permission from that person is just plain rude and ethically wrong.

2. Because working in a coning is a physical phenomenon for us, we need to address some basic physical needs.

a) Normally, we should not work in a coning for more than *one hour at a time.* This is especially true in the beginning when we are getting used to working with and in a coning. Your body needs time to adjust to this new dynamic. If you need to do more than can be accomplished within the one-hour time frame, close down the coning and continue in a new coning later that day or the next day.

b) Activating, working with, and dismantling a coning require sharp focus on our part. As a result, we may experience a protein drain. You will know you are experiencing such a drain if you come out of the coning and are suddenly attacked with a galloping case of the munchies. Often, we translate a protein drain into a desire for sweets. I have nothing against a great big piece of chocolate from time to time. But in this case, you need protein to compensate for the drain. Then eat your chocolate.

HINT: Have a bag of nuts with you while you are in a coning and occasionally down a few. This will avoid or minimize the protein drain while you are in the coning.

Also, I find that while in the coning, I do not perceive the protein drain or any hunger. It doesn't register until after I close down the coning. So I suggest that, if you are not hungry during the coning, don't let that fool you. Still have your supply of nuts handy, and eat a few throughout the session.

3. If you need to take a break during a coning session, do not close the coning and then re-open it. Just tell your team that you need a break for fifteen minutes or a half-hour or whatever (don't make it a vacation). They will automatically shift the coning into what I call the "at-rest" position. You may feel the intensity of the coning back off a bit when this shift occurs. It will take about five seconds. Then have your break. When you are ready to resume, announce that your break is over and that you would like to fully activate the coning again, and the coning will automatically shift back into its previous connection and intensity.

4. Don't get into the habit of activating conings indiscriminately. They are to be used for interlevel work and process, and not for prediction-type information. Your coning members are functioning in a teamlike dynamic with you and do not wish to be asked to function in areas where your common sense should be the dominant factor. Opening a coning to ask if you should go on a specific vacation or if it would be good for you to invest money in a certain stock is not appropriate. As far as your team is concerned, such decisions are best left to your common sense and intelligence.

I also suggest that you limit the questions to issues that pertain to the present. Information about the future is reliable only if *all* issues and elements involved remain *exactly* the same as they were when you asked your questions. In a changing world populated by people with active free wills, this never happens. By the time you get to some future point in time, all issues and elements will most likely have changed perspective and position. Therefore your answers about what to do will also need to change. In short, it is a waste of time and a crapshoot to try to see into the future—from within a coning or otherwise.

There is something else I would like to explain. Many people use kinesiology to discern issues about themselves. For example, they may wish to know if they are to take a certain vitamin. This is a question that can be accurately answered using kinesiology and should not be addressed in a coning. If I want to know whether I should wear yellow or red for a special occasion in order to enhance my strength and balance, *my* electrical system has the answer. Either my electrical system is strong when I hold that color or it is weak. A simple kinesiology test will accurately discern this for me. I don't need to call a team meeting.

Appendix B

Kinesiology

I have mentioned that one of the best and most effective means for communicating with a White Brotherhood Medical Team or in any coning is kinesiology. Kinesiology is a fancy name for muscle testing. If you want to get medical information from your team, all you have to do is ask simple yes/no questions that will cover the information you seek. (By "simple," I mean questions that can have only one answer, not two questions in one sentence, each requiring its own answer.) Your team will project a yes or no into your electrical system and you will then be able to discern their answer by kinesiology. For those of you who already use this method for getting information from nature or for testing the essences, you already have the tool in place for communicating with your team. Just direct your questions to them. But make sure the questions are in the *simple* yes/no format. And do the kinesiology test.

For those of you who have never heard of such a thing but would like to try it, I am reprinting the information on developing kinesiology testing from the books, *Flower Essences* and *Perelandra Garden Workbook: Second Edition.*

KINESIOLOGY:
THE TOOL FOR TESTING

Kinesiology is simple. Anybody can do it because it uses your electrical system and your muscles. If you are alive, you have these two things. I know that sounds smart-mouthed of me, but I've learned that sometimes people refuse to believe anything can be so simple. So they create a mental block—only "sensitive types" can do this, or only women can do this. It's just not true. Kinesiology happens to be one of those simple things in life just waiting around to be learned and used by everyone.

I don't mean to intimidate you, but small children can learn to do kinesiology in about five minutes. It is mainly because it never occurred to them that they couldn't do it. If I tell them they have an electrical system, they don't argue with me about it—they just get on with the business of learning how to do simple testing. Actually, I do mean to intimidate you. Your first big hurdle will be whether or not you believe you have a viable electrical system that is capable of being tested. Here's a good test. Place a hand mirror under your nose. If you see breath marks, you have a strong electrical system. (If you don't see breath marks, you probably no longer need MAP.) Now you can get on with learning how to test!

If you've ever been to a chiropractor or wholistic physician experienced in muscle testing, you've experienced kinesiology. The doctor tells you to stick out your arm and resist his pressure. It feels like he is trying to push your arm down after he has told you not to let him do it. Everything is going fine, and then all of a sudden he presses and your arm falls down like a floppy fish. That is using kinesiology.

Simply stated, the body has within it and surrounding it an electrical network or grid. If a negative energy (that is, any physical object or energy vibration that does not maintain or enhance health and balance) is introduced into a person's overall energy field, his muscles, when having physical pressure applied, are unable to hold their strength. (The ablility to hold muscle power is directly linked to the balance of the electrical system.) In other words, if pressure is applied to an individual's extended arm while his field is affected by a negative (energy), the arm will not be able to resist the pressure. It will weaken and fall to his side. If pressure is applied while affected by a positive (energy), the person will easily resist and the arm will hold its position. In MAP, the team answers your yes/no questions by projecting a positive energy or negative energy—whichever is appropriate—into your electrical system. The yes or no you receive in the testing is actually from your team's projected answer. It is not an answer that has been concocted by you.

In kinesiology, when a negative is placed within a person's energy field, his electrical system will immediately respond by short-circuiting or overloading. This makes it difficult, if not impossible, for the muscles to maintain their strength and hold the position when any pressure is added. When a positive is within a person's energy field, the electrical system holds, and the muscles maintain their strength when pressure is applied.

This electrical/muscular relationship is a natural part of the human system. It is not mystical or magical. Kinesiology is the established method for reading that balance at any given moment.

If you have ever experienced muscle testing, you most likely participated in the above-described, two-person operation. You provided the extended arm, and the other person provided the pressure. Although efficient, this can sometimes be cumbersome when you want to test something on your own. Arm pumpers have the nasty habit of disappearing right when you need them most. So you will be learning to self-test—no arm pumpers needed.

KINESIOLOGY SELF-TESTING STEPS

1. THE CIRCUIT FINGERS. *If you are right-handed:* Place your left hand palm up. Connect the tip of your left thumb with the tip of the left little finger (*not your index finger*). *If you are left-handed:* Place your right hand palm up. Connect the tip of your right thumb with the tip of your right little finger. By connecting your thumb and little finger, you have just closed an electrical circuit in your hand, and it is this circuit you will use for testing.

Before going on, look at the position you have just formed with your hand. If your thumb is touching the tip of your index or first finger, laugh at yourself for not being able to follow directions, and change the position to touch the tip of the thumb with the tip of the little or fourth finger. Most likely this will not feel at all comfortable to you. If you are feeling a weird sense of awkwardness, you've got the first step of the test position! In time, the hand and fingers will adjust to being put in this position and it will feel fine.

Circuit fingers can touch tip to tip, finger pad to finger pad, or thumbnail resting on top of little finger's nail. Women with long nails need not impale themselves.

2. THE TEST FINGERS. To test the circuit (the means by which you will apply pressure to yourself), place the

thumb and index finger of your other hand inside the circle you have created by connecting your thumb and little finger. The thumb/index finger should be right under the thumb/little finger, touching them. Don't try to make a circle with your test fingers. They are just placed inside the circuit fingers that do form a circle. It will look as if the circuit fingers are resting on the test fingers.

3. POSITIVE RESPONSE. Keeping this position, ask yourself a yes/no question in which you already know the answer to be yes. ("Is my name _____?") Once

you've asked the question, press your circuit fingers together, keeping the tip-to-tip position. *Using the same amount of pressure,* try to push apart the circuit fingers with your test fingers. Press the lower thumb against the upper thumb, the lower index finger against the upper little finger.

The action of your test fingers will look like scissors separating as you try separating your circuit fingers. The motion of the test fingers is horizontal. Don't try to pull your test fingers vertically up through your circuit fingers. This action sometimes works but it is not as reliable as the horizontal scissors action.

The circuit position described in step 1 corresponds to the position you take when you stick your arm out for the physician. The testing position in step 2 is in place of a physician or other convenient arm pumper. After you ask the yes/no question and you press your circuit fingers tip-to-tip, that is equal to the doctor saying, "Resist my pressure." Your circuit fingers now correspond to your outstretched, stiffened arm. Trying to push apart those fingers with your testing fingers is equal to the doctor pressing down on your arm.

If the answer to the question is positive (if your name is what you think it is!), you will not be able to easily pull apart the circuit fingers. The electrical circuit will hold, your muscles will maintain their strength, and your circuit fingers will not separate. You will feel the strength in that circuit. *IMPORTANT: Be sure the amount of pressure holding the circuit fingers together is equal to the amount of your testing fingers pressing against them. Also, don't use a pumping action in your test fingers when trying to pry your circuit fingers apart. Use an equal, steady, and continuous pressure.*

Play with this a bit. Ask a few more yes/no questions that have positive answers. Now, I know it is going to seem that if you already know the answer to be yes, you are probably "throwing" the test. That's reasonable, but for the time being, until you get a feeling for what the positive response feels like, you're going to need to deliberately ask yourself questions with positive answers.

While asking questions, if you are having trouble sensing the strength of the circuit, apply a little more pressure. Or consider that you may be applying too much pressure and pull back some. You don't have to break or strain your fingers for this; just use enough pressure to make them feel alive, connected, and alert.

4. NEGATIVE RESPONSE. Once you have a clear sense of the positive response, ask yourself a question that has a negative answer. Again press your circuit fingers together and, *using equal pressure*, press against the circuit fingers with the test fingers. This time the electrical circuit will break and the circuit fingers will weaken and separate. Because the electrical circuit is broken, the muscles in the circuit fingers do not have the power to

hold the fingers together. In a
positive state the electrical circuit
holds, and the muscles have the
power to keep the two fingers
together.

How much your circuit fingers
separate depends on your personal style. Some people's fingers
separate a lot. Other's barely separate at all. Mine
separate about a quarter of an inch. Some people's
fingers won't separate at all, but they'll definitely feel
the fingers weaken when pressure is applied during a no
answer. Let your personal style develop naturally.

Also, if you are having a little trouble feeling anything, do your testing with your forearms resting in
your lap. This way you won't be using your muscles to
hold up your arms while trying to test.

Play with negative questions a bit, and then return to
positive questions. Get a good feeling for the strength
between your circuit fingers when the electricity is in a
positive state and the weakness when the electricity is in
a negative state. You can even ask yourself (your own
system) for a positive response and then, after testing,
ask for a negative response. ("Give me a positive
response." Test. "Give me a negative response." Test.)
You will feel the positive strength and the negative
weakness. In the beginning, you may feel only a slight
difference between the two. With practice, that difference
will become more pronounced. For now, it is just a matter of trusting what you have learned—and practicing.

Don't forget the overall concept behind kinesiology. What enhances our body, mind, and soul makes us strong. Together, our body, mind, and soul create a wholistic environment that, when balanced, is strong and solid. If something enters that environment and negates or challenges the balance, the environment is weakened. That strength or weakness registers in the electrical system, and it can be discerned through the muscle-testing technique—kinesiology.

KINESIOLOGY TIPS

If you are having trouble feeling the electrical circuit in the circuit fingers, try switching hands—the circuit fingers become the test fingers and vice versa. Most people who are right-handed have this particular electrical circuitry in their left hand. Left-handers generally have the circuitry in their right hand. But sometimes a right-hander has the circuitry in the right hand and a left-hander has it in the left hand. You may be one of those people. If you are ambidextrous, choose the circuit hand that gives you the clearest responses. Before deciding which to use, give yourself a couple of weeks of testing using one hand as the circuit hand to get a good feel for its responses before trying the other hand.

If you have an injury such as a muscle sprain in either hand or arm, don't try to learn kinesiology until you have healed. Kinesiology is *muscle* testing, and a muscle injury will interfere with the testing—and the testing will interfere with the healing of the muscle injury.

Also, when first learning kinesiology, do yourself a favor and set aside some quiet time to go through the instructions and play with the testing. Trying to learn this while riding the New York subway during evening rush hour isn't going to give you the break you need. But once you have learned it, you will be able to test all kinds of things while riding the subway.

Sometimes I meet people who are trying to learn kinesiology and aren't having much luck. They've gotten frustrated, decided this isn't for them, and have gone on to try to learn another means of testing. Well, I'll listen to them explain what they did, and before they know it, I've verbally tricked them with a couple of suggestions about their testing, which they try, and they begin feeling kinesiology for the first time—a strong "yes" and a clear "no." The problem wasn't kinesiology. Everyone, as I have said, has an electrical system. The problem was that they wanted to learn it so much that they became overly anxious and tense—they blocked.

So, since you won't have me around to trick you, I suggest that if you suspect you're blocking, go on to something else. Then trick yourself. When you care the least about whether or not you learn kinesiology, start playing with it again. Approach it as if it were a game. *Then* you'll feel the strength and weakness in the fingers.

If you're still not getting a satisfactory yes and no after several weeks of trying, ask your MAP team to help you learn and develop kinesiology. You may have such a mental block around learning kinesiology that you might need a MAP/Calibration to unjam the logs around this issue.

Now, suppose the testing has been working fine, and then suddenly you can't get a clear result (what I call a "definite maybe") or get no result at all. Check:

1. Sloppy testing. You try to press apart the fingers *before* applying pressure between the circuit fingers. This happens especially when we've been testing for awhile and become over-confident or do the testing very quickly. I think it happens to all of us from time to time and serves to remind us to keep our attention on the matter at hand. (Excuse the pun.)

Especially in the beginning, start a kinesiology session by first feeling a few positive and negative responses. Ask yourself some of those obvious questions. Or simply say several times, "Let me feel a positive." (Test.) "Let me feel a negative." (Test.) This will serve as a kind of warm-up, and remind you what positive and negative feel like before you start.

2. External distractions. Trying to test in a noisy or active area can cause you to lose concentration. The testing will feel unsure or contradict itself if you double-check the results. Often, simply moving to a quiet, calm spot and concentrating on what you are doing will be just what's needed for successful testing.

3. Focus or concentration. Even in a quiet spot, one's mind may wander and the testing will feel fuzzy, weak,

or contradictory. It is important to concentrate through-out the process. Check how you are feeling. If you're tired, I suggest you not try to test until you have rested a bit. And if you have to go to the bathroom, do it. That little situation is a sure concentration-destroyer.

4. The question isn't clear. A key to kinesiology is asking a *simple* yes/no question, not two questions in one, each having a possible yes/no answer. If your testing isn't working, first check your hand positions. Next, review your question, and make sure you are asking only one question. And, while you're asking a question, don't think ahead to the next question! Your fingers won't know which to answer.

5. Match your intent with how you word your question. If you are prone to saying, "Oh, I didn't mean to say that!" when you talk to others, this might be an area you need to work on.

A woman at one of our workshops asked me about some strange answers she had gotten about what to feed her cat. She had asked, "What kinds of food would make my cat happy?" She got weird answers like chocolate, catnip, steak.... I pointed out that she probably asked the wrong question. She meant to ask what foods would make her cat *healthy*. She was a little surprised. She thought that this was the question she had originally asked. In short, her question and her intent didn't match.

6. You must want to accept the results of the test. If

you enter a kinesiology test not wanting to "hear" the answer, for whatever reason, you can override the test with your emotions and your will. This is true for conventional situations as well. If you really don't want something to work for you, it won't work. That's our personal power dictating the outcome.

Also, if you are trying to do testing during a situation that is especially emotional for you, that deeply stirs your emotions, or if you are trying to ask a question in which you have a strong, personal investment in the answer—such as, "Should I buy this beautiful $250,000 house?"—I suggest that you not test until you are calmer or get some emotional distance from the situation. During such times, you are walking a very fine line between a clear test and a test that your desires are overriding. Kinesiology as a tool is not the issue here. It is the condition or intent of the tester. In fact, some questions just shouldn't be asked, but *which questions* are relative to who is doing the asking. We each need to develop discernment around which questions are *appropriate* for us to ask.

When I am involved with testing during emotionally stressful times, I stop for a moment, collect my thoughts, and make a commitment to concentrate on the testing only. If I need to test an emotionally charged question or a question about something I have a personal investment in, I stop a moment, commit myself to the test and open myself to receiving *the* answer and not the answer I might desire.

IMPORTANT: I suggest that you make it a rule not to

ask questions like, "Do I have AIDS?" in your MAP sessions. Your ability to perceive the answer either through kinesiology or inner hearing is questionable. It is too emotionally charged. If you have a suspicion, get a solid diagnosis from the allopathic medical establishment, and make sure you get two or three "second opinions." But continue working with your MAP team throughout the diagnosis process.

7. If your testing has been going along just fine and you suddenly begin to get contradictory or "mushy" test results, consider that this may not be a good day for you to do this particular work. Or you may need to drink water. If you are dehydrated, your electrical system will feel weak during kinesiology testing. Or you may need to test yourself for flower essences. The essences balance and repair the electrical system, and this may be just what you need for clear kinesiology results.

A NOTE ON CLARITY

If you are having difficulty wording a simple yes/no question, consider this an important issue to be faced and something worth spending time to rectify. You have not simply stumbled upon a glitch in your quest to use kinesiology. You have also stumbled upon a glitch in the communication between your higher self and your conscious self. If you can't even clearly phrase the question, you can't expect an answer. I have met people who cannot articulate a question. In a workshop they will attempt to ask me something and I can't figure out what they are asking—nor can anyone else in the workshop. Usually it turns out that they are frustrated because they can't get any clarity in their own life and are trying to ask me what to do about it.

For those of you who find yourselves in this boat, you have a terrific opportunity to turn that around and develop internal order by learning how to articulate a simple yes/no question. If you do this, you not only develop the tool of kinesiology, you also develop clarity for communicating with yourself. I fully understand that it will take focus on your part, and in comparison to someone who finds articulating a simple question easy, to you it will seem herculean. But if you wish to function consciously on your many levels, you must have internal clarity and order.

I recommend that you initially devote your attention to learning to ask simple questions and not worry about receiving answers. When you need to ask someone a question, take time to consider what you really want to ask and how it can be most clearly and efficiently worded. It helps to write down the question. In this way, you can visually see your words. If they don't convey what you mentally want to express, play with the wording. Keep doing this until you feel those words accurately and concisely communicate what you wish to ask. Then go to that person and ask the question. Notice the difference in the quality of how the person answers you. Your clarity will inspire similar clarity in the response.

I urge you to continue this process for a fair period of

time—even dedicating yourself to the process for a year. Quite often, that frustrating inner confusion exists because we have not had an acceptable framework for the development of mental ordering. Learning to ask questions gives the mind something tangible to work with and, in the process, you learn mind-word-and-mouth coordination. You'll find that as you develop the ability to clearly articulate a question, your inner fog will begin to lift, which in turn will automatically begin to lift your outer fog.

Another point about clarity: As you develop internal order, your intuition will become clearer and stronger. You will see that when you ask a simple yes/no question, you will intuitively sense the answer or begin to hear your team answer before testing. This is a normal development. I recommend that you continue with the kinesiology testing as a verification that your intuitive or "overheard" answer is correct.

It is also helpful, especially in the beginning, to literally verbalize your questions out loud and not just think them. When we say something aloud, we tend to articulate it better than when we just think it. And I will ask something out loud if I'm a little tired and I need some extra sensory input (sound) to help me keep my focus.

FINAL COMMENTS ON KINESIOLOGY

Kinesiology is like any tool. The more you practice, the better you become at using it. You need a sense of confidence about using this tool, especially when you get some very strange answers to what you thought were pretty straight questions. It helps you get over the initial "this-is-weird-and-the-damned-testing-isn't-working" stage if you have some confidence in your ability to feel clear positive and negative responses. The only way I know to get over this hump is to practice testing. You will develop clarity in your testing and you'll learn your personal pitfalls.

In teaching kinesiology, I have found that something interesting happens to some people when they are learning it. Every block, doubt, question, and personal challenge they have, when faced head-on with something perceived as unconventional, comes right to the surface. It is as if the physical tool of kinesiology itself serves to bring to the surface all those hurdles. So they learn kinesiology right away and are using it well. Then, all of a sudden it is not working for them. When they tell me about it, I realize that the thing they do differently now that they didn't do at first is double-checking their answers—and rechecking, and rechecking, and doing it again, and again. . . . Each time the answers vary or the fingers get mushy and they get definite maybe's.

Well, again the issue is not the kinesiology. The issue is really why they are suddenly doing all this rechecking business. What has surfaced for them are questions

around trust in their own ability, belief that such unconventional things really do happen and are happening to
them. They have a sudden lack of self-confidence.

Again, the only way I know to get over this hurdle is
to defy it—keep testing. The other alternative is to suc-
cumb and stop developing kinesiology. But, that doesn't
really accomplish anything. So in cases like this, I suggest the person keep testing, *stop* double-checking and
take the plunge to go with the first test result. Eventually, what action is taken based on the first test result will
verify the accuracy of the test. From this, your confidence builds. I firmly believe that only clear personal
experience and evidence can get us through these kinds
of hurdles and blocks—and that means just continuing
to go on.

So, what can we practice-test on? Everything. You
could easily drive yourself nuts. What colors you should
wear. What colors you should wear for a special event.
What would be healthiest for you to eat for breakfast,
lunch, and dinner. You take ten separate vitamin and
mineral supplements as a matter of course on a daily
basis. Try testing them individually ("Do I need vitamin
E? B6? Iron?") to see if you need all ten everyday. Or
test to see if there are some you don't need to take at all.
You are sitting at a restaurant and they don't have Tofu
Supreme on the menu. Is there anything on that menu
that is healthy for you to eat? ("Should I eat fish?"
[yes/no] "Should I eat beef?" [yes/no] "Chicken?"
[yes/no] "Häagen-Dazs fudge ripple ice cream?" [yes!])

And one thing you can frequently test yourself for is whether or not you need flower essences.

The point is to test everything you possibly can that doesn't place you in a life-threatening situation, follow through on your answers, and then look at the results. As I have worked through the years to refine my ability to use kinesiology, I have, on many occasions, purposely followed through on answers that made no sense at all to me, just to see if the testing was accurate. Doing this and looking at the results with a critical eye is the only way I know to learn about ourselves as kinesiology testers and to discover the nuances and uses of kinesiology itself.

One last piece of information: Give yourself about a year to develop a strong confidence with kinesiology. Now, you'll be able to use it right away. This just takes sticking with your initial efforts until you get those first feelings of positive strength and negative weakness in the circuit fingers. But I have found from my own experience and from watching others that it takes about a year of experimentation to fully learn the art of asking accurate yes/no questions and to overcome the hurdles. As one woman said, "You stick with this stuff a year, and boy, what a great thing you end up with!"

Appendix C

Flower Essences

For those of you who would like to know more about flower essences, I am reprinting the section on flower essences from the Perelandra Catalog. As part of the co-creative garden work here at Perelandra, we produce five sets of flower essences: Perelandra Rose Essences, Perelandra Garden Essences, Perelandra Rose Essences II, Perelandra Nature Program Essences, and the Perelandra Soul Ray Essences. There are a number of flower essences available in the United States, Australia, and Great Britain, and it is unimportant to me and to MAP which essences you use—as long as the are the ones you are most comfortable with. So I offer you the Perelandra information in the spirit of giving you general information about flower essences and specific information about the Perelandra Essences. In this Appendix is a short list of other flower essence suppliers who will be happy to send you their catalogs on request.

The human body has within and surrounding it an electrical network. When we experience health, this electrical network is balanced and fully connected. When something in our life or environment threatens that balance, the electrical system responds by either short-circuiting or overloading. That imbalance in the electrical system immediately impacts the central nervous system. The body then goes into high gear in an effort to correct the imbalance. If our body does not succeed, we physically manifest the imbalance. We get a cold or a headache, or our allergy pops up again or another migraine belts us. Or we get back pain, or our neck goes out again. Or we become seriously ill.

Flower essences work directly with both the electrical and the central nervous systems. By taking the correct essences, we immediately balance the electrical system, stabilize the nervous system, and stop the domino effect that leads to illness.

If we don't take flower essences and wind up getting sick, we can still take the essence(s) that will then stabilize and balance the electrical and nervous systems while the body gets on with the business of fighting off the problem. By assisting this process, flower essences drastically reduce our recovery time. In short, by using the essences, we are not asking our body to pull double duty—to do the work to heal us systemically *and* rebalance our electrical and central nervous systems.

A different perspective about the essences, excerpted from a session with the Deva of Flower Essences might be helpful:

You are getting the idea that all is changing. How one perceives his health is also changing. As with everything around him, the key to this change is balance. One's health will be intimately linked with one's understanding and response to balance.

. . . Flower essences support and help secure balance on all levels—physical, emotional, mental, and spiritual. Physically, they balance the body by reconnecting and adjusting the electrical system. Emotionally and mentally, they help the person identify, alter, and sometimes remove emotional and mental patterns that challenge overall balance. And spiritually, they assist the person's connection to and understanding of the many levels of self to be able to operate in life from a broader perspective.

Flower essences provide a health system that is aligned to both the surrounding universal dynamics of transition, and the individual's expansion and response to the times by having incorporated within the system itself the key to it all—balance.

The Perelandra Rose and Garden Essences have been a natural development in the work that has gone on between nature and myself. They are produced from the flowers, vegetables, and herbs grown in the Perelandra garden. These essences are carefully prepared and stabilized pattern-infused water tinctures that are then preserved in brandy. The tinctures go through a final stabilization inside the genesa crystal sitting in the center of the garden. They are bottled in concentrate form in pharmaceutical dropper bottles that make it easy and convenient for you to place one drop of a needed essence directly on your tongue or several drops of the essence in a glass of water to be sipped throughout the day.

I feel that through these flower essences we at Perelandra are able to share the extraordinary vitality and power that has resulted from our co-creative work with nature in the Perelandra garden. In using the essences, we establish another partnership with nature—this one focused on our health, balance, and well-being.

If you are intrigued, interested, or curious about flower essences and wish to investigate them further, I offer some suggestions on how you might proceed without feeling overwhelmed.

❋ Read *Flower Essences: Reordering Our Understanding and Approach to Illness and Health.* It will give you a crystal-clear idea about what flower essences are, the testing techniques and processes used, how to choose the essences you need, and suggestions on how to successfully integrate them into your life. The Perelandra essences are fully discussed, but the book is applicable to all flower essences and presents step-by-step processes that can be used for any essences on the market. (If you already have a set of essences and wish to use them with greater effectiveness and precision, you might consider getting the book *Flower Essences.*)

❋ For those who would like to try essences and experience how they work: Read through the Perelandra essence definitions that are listed in this appendix. Then think about some physical, emotional, mental, or spiritual problem you would like to address. Think of it clearly or even write it out. Then say to yourself, "What essence(s) do I need to help me with this problem now?"

Read through the definitions again and note which one(s) *intuitively* pop out to you. (If you know kinesiology, you can simply test the list of essences, choosing the ones that test positive for you.) Order the essences that stand out when you read the definitions. (Try to keep your rational mind out of the process!) You'll get a Guide with the bottles that will explain how to use them and teach you how to find out how often to take them. Usually one drop, once or twice daily for several days, will do the trick. Then see how you feel. Also, get the book *Flower Essences* so that you can see more clearly when and how they are to be used.

✳ For those, like myself, who are immediately struck between the eyes by these things called "flower essences" and know they belong in your life: I strongly suggest that you purchase the **Basic Set** of Perelandra Essences—that is, both the **Rose Essences (Set I)** and the **Garden Essences**. This is an excellent starter combination for day-to-day process and issues. Now, to be honest with you, I've been reluctant to suggest this to people. I'm sensitive to the fact that we're talking about money here and, as the producer/developer of the Perelandra essences, there is an obvious conflict of interest in my suggestion. But I feel urged to come out of the closet with this suggestion for three reasons:

1. These two sets often work in *combination* with one another. The Rose Essences address and support the various steps of the process we move through as we face daily challenge and change. The Garden Essences

address specific issues on the physical, emotional, mental, and spiritual levels that either trigger transition or arise because of it. In my work as an essence practitioner, I have found that often a person needs support for both the daily transition process itself and the specific issues coming up due to the process.

2. The Basic Set of Perelandra Essences covers a wide range of transition and specific issues. What is needed this week will often be different from what is needed next week or next month or next year. The essences are used one or two drops at a time and have an indefinite shelf life. In short, you'll be keeping and using the set for many years. It is fair to assume that you or someone close to you will be needing each of the essences at some point. It is more convenient to have them on hand when needed rather than have to order those specific bottles and wait for them to arrive in the mail before using them.

3. I have noticed over the years that a fair number of people initially ordering single bottles or partial sets end up ordering the Basic Set. After using them, they came to the conclusion that to use the essences with the greatest agility and accuracy, one needs to have on hand the wide range provided by the Basic Set of Perelandra Essences.

I also suggest that when ordering the Basic Set of Perelandra Essences, you include *Flower Essences* along with your order. I know I am suggesting this book a lot. But I feel strongly that it will help you to organize and integrate the essences into your life in a precise and extremely effective manner.

Expanded Set of Perelandra Essences: In 1992 we developed a third set of flower essences: **Perelandra Rose Essences II.** This set of eight essences balances and stabilizes the body's central nervous system. They also address the balancing needs of our central nervous system that are activated and/or impacted during a deep expansion experience. These experiences, by their nature, require that we address and integrate something completely new and, as a result, we change our personal and world view. Here, one is not processing ordinary, everyday occurrences. Rather, one is faced with an experience that challenges the central nervous system's capability to balance and function. From the response we have from flower essences folks to this set, it seems that nearly everyone is testing for Rose II a lot. If you are interested in incorporating flower essences into your life, I suggest that you purchase the Expanded Set—that is, the Perelandra Rose and Garden Essences plus Rose Essences II.

With each purchase—individual bottles or sets—you also get the beginner's Guide that gives the step-by-step basic processes for testing yourself for the essences you need and the correct dosage (i.e., how many drops of the essences are needed for how many days). Also included in the Guide are long definitions for each of the essences. Reading them will give you a clearer idea of what the essences address.

Perelandra Rose Essences (Set I)

The Perelandra Rose Essences are a set of eight flower essences. Made from roses in the Perelandra garden, these eight essences function with one another to support and balance an individual as he proceeds in day-to-day evolutionary process. As we move forward in daily process, there are mechanisms within us that are set in motion to facilitate our periods of growth. The Perelandra Rose Essences help stabilize and balance us and our process mechanisms.

The following are short definitions of the Perelandra Rose Essences. The name of each essence is the same as the rose from which it is made.

GRUSS AN AACHEN: Stability. Balances and stabilizes the body/soul unit on all PEMS levels (physical, emotional, mental, spiritual) as it moves forward in its evolutionary process.

PEACE: Courage. Opens the individual to the inner dynamic of courage that is aligned to universal courage.

ECLIPSE: Acceptance and insight. Enhances the individual's appreciation of his own inner knowing. Supports the mechanism that allows the body to receive the soul's input and insight.

ORANGE RUFFLES: Receptivity. Stabilizes the individual during the expansion of his sensory system.

AMBASSADOR: Pattern. Aids the individual in seeing

270

the relationship of the part to the whole, in perceiving his pattern and purpose.

NYMPHENBURG: Strength. Supports and holds the strength created by the balance of the body/soul fusion, and facilitates the individual's ability to regain that balance.

WHITE LIGHTNIN': Synchronized movement. Stabilizes the inner timing of all PEMS levels moving in concert, and enhances the body/soul fusion.

ROYAL HIGHNESS: Final stabilization. The mop-up essence that helps to insulate, protect, and stabilize the individual and to stabilize the shift during its final stages while the individual is vulnerable.

Perelandra Garden Essences

This set of eighteen essences is made from the flower petals of vegetables, herbs, and flowers grown in the Perelandra garden. Their balancing and restorative patterns address physical, emotional, mental, and spiritual issues that we face in today's world.

BROCCOLI: For the power balance that must be maintained when one perceives himself to be under siege from outside. Stabilizes the body/soul unit so the person won't close down, detach, and scatter.

CAULIFLOWER: Stabilizes and balances the child during the birth process. Stabilizes body/soul balance in adults.

CELERY: Restores balance of the immune system when it is being overworked or stressed, and during long-term viral or bacterial infections.

CHIVES: Re-establishes the power one has when the internal male/female dynamics are balanced, and the person is functioning in a state of awareness within this balance.

COMFREY: Repairs higher vibrational soul damage that occurred in the present or a past lifetime.

CORN: Stabilization during universal/spiritual expansion. Assists transition of experience into useful, pertinent understanding and action.

CUCUMBER: Rebalancing during depression. Vital reattachment to life.

DILL: Assists individual in reclaiming power balance one has released to others. Releases victimization.

NASTURTIUM: Restores vital physical life energy during times of intense mental-level focus.

OKRA: Returns ability to see the positive in one's life and environment.

SALVIA: Restores emotional stability during times of extreme stress.

SNAP PEA: Rebalances child or adult after a nightmare. Assists in ability to translate daily experience into positive, understandable process.

SUMMER SQUASH: Restores courage to the person who experiences fear and resistance when faced with daily routine. Releases shyness and phobia issues.

SWEET BELL PEPPER: Restores inner peace, clarity, and calm when faced with stressful times. Stabilizes body/soul balance during times of stress.

TOMATO: Cleansing. Assists the body in shattering and throwing off that which is causing infection or disease.

YELLOW YARROW: Supplies emotional protection during vulnerable times. Its support softens resistance and assists the integration process.

ZINNIA: Reconnects one to the child within. Restores playfulness, laughter, joy, and a sense of healthy priorities.

ZUCCHINI: Helps restore physical strength during convalescence.

Perelandra Rose Essences II

This set of Perelandra flower essences was developed in 1992. The eight essences are made from roses growing in the Perelandra garden and address the specific balancing and stabilizing needs of the body's central nervous system. They also address the functions within the central nervous system that are activated and/or impacted during a *deep expansion experience*. Here, one is not simply processing ordinary, everyday occurrences. Rather, one is faced with an experience that is new and

273

challenging to the present balance and functioning of the body. When faced with this kind of expansion, the central nervous system is required to function in new ways, and with patterns and rhythms yet to be experienced. The Rose Essences II address this phenomenon by balancing and stabilizing this system's functions that have been impacted by the expansion.

I wish I could list specific experiences that would identify deep expansion situations for you, but a deep expansion for some is an everyday life process for others. The only thing I can say is that if you are interested in Perelandra, MAP, and incorporating flower essences in your life, you are the kind of person who doesn't shy away from deep expansion. I think it would be good to have this set of handy.

The following are the short definitions for Rose II. The name of each essence is the same as the name of the rose from which it is made.

BLAZE IMPROVED CLIMBING ROSE: Softens and relaxes first the central nervous system and then the body as a whole, thus allowing the input from an expansion experience to be appropriately sorted, shifted, and integrated within the body.

MAYBELLE STEARNS: Stabilizes and supports the sacrum during an expansion experience.

MR. LINCOLN: Balances and stabilizes the cerebrospinal fluid (CSF) pulse while it alters its rhythm and patterning to accommodate the expansion.

SONIA: Stabilizes and supports the CSF pulse *after* it has completed its shift to accommodate the expansion.

CHICAGO PEACE: Stabilizes movement of and interaction among the cranial bones, CSF, and sacrum during an expansion experience.

BETTY PRIOR: Stabilizes and balances the delicate rhythm of expansion and contraction of the cranial bones during the expansion.

TIFFANY: Stabilizes the cranials as they shift their alignment appropriately to accommodate the input and impulses of expansion.

OREGOLD: Stabilizes and balances the cranials, central nervous system, CSF, and sacrum after an expansion process is complete.

Perelandra Nature Program Essences

This is an exciting development for us. The Perelandra Nature Program Essences are the next step in developing our understanding of health and electrical-system balancing. These essences are groundbreaking in that, by working in partnership with nature, the elements that are used as the foundation for the creation of these essences literally span the globe.

Another groundbreaking aspect of these essences is that the balancing pattern each essence contains is not present in any single element or combination of elements on the planet. These are new patterns devically created to address the complexity of today's health issues. Although each essence has as its foundation a combination of patterns from existing elements found around the globe, when combined on the devic level (as in this essence production process), the various patterns create a chemical-like explosion that results in a single, entirely new pattern that is not available anywhere else on the planet. New balancing patterns have been created for this set of essences without having to create new plant varieties or other natural elements for holding these patterns.

The major dynamic of these essences centers around the concept of balance. In balance there is automatic healing. An organism cannot be in balance and at the same time be in need of healing. Consequently, these essences focus on shifting to appropriate balance the internal environment of any living organism (such as the internal environment of the human body) and its relationship with the larger external environment. With the six V, F, and B essences, the focus is on achieving an appropriate internal balance that will automatically adjust a viral, fungal, or bacterial imbalance. The Sobopla, Moon, and Bowl essences address the balance of a living organism within the larger picture.

All living organisms relate to and interact with viruses, fungi, and bacteria both within the organism's internal environment (its body) and within the surrounding, larger environment. Balance implies that their presence has a harmonious effect on the organism. Problems arise when imbalance within the organism occurs, thus causing an imbalance with any specific combination of viruses, fungi, or bacteria. As a result, the organism develops health problems that have as their root cause a fungal, viral and/or bacterial imbalance.

The V, F, and B essences do not approach an imbalanced, problematic situation from the perspective of eradicating virus, fungus, and/or bacteria. They restore internal environmental balance and the balanced existence of the specific viruses, fungi, and/or bacteria found within that environment. As a result, you have a vibrant, balanced living organism that includes an appropriate relationship and interaction with existing and surrounding viruses, fungi, and bacteria. You will find that when you address health issues from the perspective of balancing all the various elements involved, you will be restoring a living organism to health—be it human, plant, or animal—more quickly than ever perceived possible.

NATURE PROGRAM ESSENCES

V-1, or F-1, or B-1: Restores the body's environment to balance when its imbalance is creating a corresponding viral, fungal, or bacterial imbalance. They also restore the body's environment to balance once a corresponding viral, fungal, or bacterial imbalance is present and impacting the body.

V-2, or F-2, or B-2: Restores a state of appropriate balance within the living viral, fungal, or bacterial organisms so that they may once again relate to and interact with their larger host organism (body) in an appropriately balanced and environmentally sound manner.

SOBOPLA: (So-bo'-pla) Balances and stabilizes the triangle created by the relationship and interaction between the soul, its physical body, and the planet upon which the body resides. As a result, the soul, body, and planet become one strong, fully functioning triangular unit. Sobopla also balances and stabilizes the physical seating of the body/soul unit to the planet.

MOON: Balances, stabilizes, and as a result strengthens the connections and links between specific elements within each living organism on this planet and the corresponding elements that are part of the Moon.

BOWL: Links humans and all other living organisms to the heart and soul impulses of the planet. Also synchronizes the human/living organism with the heart and soul impulses of the planet and the universe, thus supporting the evolutionary process of the human/living organism moving in tandem with the universe into the Aquarian era.

The Nature Program Essences Set works effectively when tested alone and with the other Perelandra Essences. They have an indefinite shelf life. *It is important that anyone using these essences have on hand the full set.* The Nature Program Essences include a boxed set of nine 1/2-oz. bottles, the Guide, and definitions.

Additional Essence Developments: In 1994, the Perelandra Soul Ray Essences were developed. The Soul Ray Essences include a boxed set of eight 1/2-oz. bottles, the Guide, and definitions. For a full description of this extraordinary essences set, see the Perelandra catalog.

IMPORTANT: I highly recommend that anyone in MAP also include the Nature Program and Soul Ray Essences with the Expanded Set. These two sets combined with the Expanded Set cover a full range of an individual's essence needs.

OTHER FLOWER ESSENCES SOURCES

If you would like an international list of flower essence producers, please send a self-addressed, stamped envelope to Perelandra.

Perelandra, Ltd.
P.O. Box 3603
Warrenton, VA 20188

ESSENCES PURCHASING INFORMATION
For prices and ordering information,
see the order form at the end of the book.

BASIC SET: The 26 Perelandra Rose (set I only) & Garden Essences purchased together. Available in one-dram (1/8 oz.) and half-ounce bottles.

Obviously, the 1/2-oz. set is more economical. The bottles are four times larger than those in the dram set. It consists of the 26 Perelandra Rose & Garden Essences in three boxes. It includes the beginner's Guide with full definitions, plus instructions on how to test for and use the essences. You also get a short-definitions card to tape on the inside of the lid for quick reference.

The Basic Dram Set contains the 26 Perelandra Rose & Garden Essences, the Guide, one empty dram solution bottle, and the short-definitions card in *one box* that measures about 6-by-8 inches. This is convenient if you take the essences on trips or shift them between home and office.

EXPANDED SET: Includes the Basic Set (Perelandra Rose & Garden Essences) plus the Perelandra Rose Essences II Set—34 bottles total. This combination is the most economical way to purchase the three flower essences sets. Available in 1/2-oz. and one-dram bottles.

ALL ESSENCES SET: Includes the Expanded Set (Perelandra Rose, Garden & Rose Essences II in dram or 1/2-oz. bottles) plus the Perelandra Nature Program and Soul Ray Essences in 1/2-oz. bottles. Each set is boxed and includes the beginner's Guide with full definitions, plus instructions on how to test the essences for yourself and others in your family. You also get a short-definitions card with each box to tape on the inside of the lid for quick reference.

PERELANDRA ROSE ESSENCES SET: (set I) Includes a box with eight 1/2-oz. *dropper bottles*, the Perelandra Essence Guide, and the short-definitions card, which may be taped to the inside of the box lid for easy reference.

PERELANDRA GARDEN ESSENCES SET: Two boxes containing a total of eighteen 1/2-oz. *dropper bottles*, the Guide, and two short-definitions cards.

PERELANDRA ROSE ESSENCES II: Includes a box with eight 1/2 oz. *dropper bottles*, the Guide, and the short-definitions card.

PERELANDRA NATURE PROGRAM ESSENCES: Includes a boxed set of nine 1/2-oz. *dropper bottles*, the Guide, and the short-definitions card.

PERELANDRA SOUL RAY ESSENCES: Includes a boxed set of eight 1/2-oz. *dropper bottles*, the Guide, and the short-definitions card.

INDIVIDUAL ESSENCES: *Half-ounce dropper bottles* plus the Guide. See the order form at the end of the book or the Perelandra catalog for details.

NOTE: If you are sensitive to brandy, you may special order your flower essences preserved in distilled white vinegar. The prices are the same. Please note your request for vinegar on the order form.

Also, the Perelandra Essences are natural and will not interfere with any medications you may be taking. However, essences are not a substitute for needed medical care.

And finally: We guarantee the integrity and potency of the Perelandra Essences. They have an indefinite shelf life and we preserve them in a brandy or vinegar base to ensure that shelf life. Sometimes, after a period of time, the rubber bulb on the dropper may show signs of deterioration—softening, collapsing, cracking. When this occurs, we recommend you replace your droppers. See the Perelandra catalog for complete details. Of course, we can't guarantee mishaps that occur due to "user carelessness," such as replacing a dropper before washing it off after it has touched your mouth or having several bottles open at one time and forgetting which dropper went into which bottle. But we certainly back the integrity of the essences in the areas that we here at Perelandra can control.

FLOWER ESSENCE TESTING

The Basic Flower Essence Test

1. Place a dropper bottle of each flower essence in your lap.

2. Ask:
Do I need any flower essences? (Test.)
If you get a negative, you're fine. Your balance is holding and you need no additional essence assistance.

3. If the result was positive, you need a flower essence. Place the bottles one by one in your lap and ask each time:
Do I need ____ essence?
The flower essence or essences that test positive are the ones you need.

4. Check your results by placing in your lap just the bottles that tested positive. Ask:
Are these the only essences I need? (Test.)
If the response is positive and you need only one bottle, go to step 5.
If you get a negative, retest the other essences. A negative means you missed an essence and need to find what was missed. After retesting, ask the question once more.
Are these the only essences I need? (Test.)
If still negative, keep testing the essences until you get a positive response to the question. This will verify to you that you have all the essences you need.

If you have more than one essence, you will need to check them as a combination by placing all of them in your lap and asking:

Is this the combination I need? (Test.)

If you get a negative even though the flower essences tested positive when tested individually, you may need to adjust the *combination*. This means that when the individual essences that tested positive were put together, a combination was created that made one or more of those essences unnecessary. The whole was stronger and more effective than the sum of its parts. Just test each of the combination bottles separately by asking:

Do I remove this bottle from the combination? (Test.)

Whatever tests positive gets removed. Then put the remaining combination bottles in your lap and ask:

Is this combination now correct? (Test.)

You should get a positive. If you don't, test the original combination again, and keep working at it until the combination tests positive as a unit.

5. Take the flower essences that you need, and then read their definitions. The easiest way to take the essences is to put one drop of each essence concentrate on your tongue, being careful not to touch your mouth with the dropper. If you do, wash the dropper well before placing it back in the bottle.

Then ask:

Am I clear? (Test.)

You should test positive at this point, and ninety-nine

times out of a hundred, you will. If you test negative, don't panic. You've already double-checked your results, so this test stands as is. A negative result means that you are ready to add an additional process, if you wish. If you would like to continue, immediately refer to the Peeling Process section in Chapter 8 of the book *Flower Essences*. This will give you the steps for continuing. However, if you do not have this book or don't wish to go on to the Peeling Process right away, test for dosage and take the flower essences for which you tested in this basic test.

Testing for Dosage

This is to find out how many days or weeks you are to take the essences you just tested for.

1. Hold all the bottles you need in your lap.

2. Ask if you need to take the flower essence(s) more than one time. If negative, that means, "No, you don't need to take them more than one time," and you have already completed the dosage by putting one drop from each bottle on your tongue.

3. If positive, you will need to find out how may days you should take the flower essences and how many times per day. Do a *sequential test*. With the needed flower essence(s) in your lap, ask yourself:
    Do I need these one day? (Test.)
    2 days? (Test.)

3 days? (Test.)

Do a count until you get a negative response. If you need the flower essences for three days, you will test positive when you ask, "1 day?", "2 days?", "3 days?" When you ask, "4 days?" you will test negative. That will tell you that your system would be assisted and strengthened by taking the flower essences for three days, not four days.

Daily Dosage

Let's say you test that you need to take the essences for three days. Now using the same format, ask if you should take the essences:

1 time daily? (Test.)

2 times daily? (Test.)

And so on, until you get a negative. Most people need to take them either one or two, sometimes three, times a day. Test until you get a negative response. Your last positive will tell you how many times per day you need to take them.

Generally, flower essences are to be taken first thing in the morning and/or last thing in the evening and/or in the mid-afternoon. If you wish to be more precise with this essence business, test to see if it is best to take them in the morning, afternoon, or evening, or any combination of the three. For example, if I am testing someone who tests for a dosage of one time a day, I always check to see if it should be in the morning, afternoon, or evening. It is usually in the morning, but I've discovered enough exceptions to that rule to test every time.

For dosages of a number of essences taken several times throughout the day over a period of days, it may be more convenient to add five drops of each needed essence to eight ounces of water (spring water or distilled water is preferred) or juice. Take one sip from this mixed solution each time you are to take the flower essences. (It is more effective if you hold the sip of solution in your mouth for a few seconds prior to swallowing.) You can store the mixture in the refrigerator. If the glass is emptied before you arc scheduled to finish taking the essences, just make the same preparation again. HINT: You can test for the precise number of drops of each essence to go into the eight ounces of water if you like. Just use the same sequential setup as was used to discover the dosage. For each essence, ask if you need:

1 drop per 8 ounces of water? (Test.)

2 drops? (Test.)

3 drops? (Test.)

And so on until you get a negative. This testing economizes to the utmost the use of your concentrates. I've suggested you use five drops per eight ounces of water because in my experience, I've never tested anyone for over five drops (most people test an average of three drops), and I figure right about now you'd appreciate a break in this testing routine.

Dosage Bottles

Suppose you need several essences several times a day, you work away from the home all day, and it's real cumbersome to transport an eight-ounce glass of water everywhere. No problem. Buy a few dropper bottles (with glass droppers) from your local pharmacy to keep on hand. Make the solution as needed right in the bottle, adding three to five drops of each essence and filling the rest of the bottle with water. (Test to see how many drops you are to use for the specific size bottle you bought.) If you are planning to use this bottle for more than a couple of days, add one teaspoon of brandy as a preservative (use more if the essences are to be taken for longer than two weeks or are exposed to high temperatures) before filling with water. Shake the dosage bottle lightly. Several flower essences may be combined in one bottle. All the essences you need for one solution should be included in the single bottle. *One dropper full*, about ten to twelve drops, from the dosage bottle can be put directly into your mouth. (Again, be careful not to touch your mouth with the dropper.)

A note on the water to be used in these solutions: Spring or untreated water is best. But if this is unavailable, tap water will suffice. You can also put the drops of essences in juice and refrigerate the solution.

A reminder: If you are sensitive to brandy, you may use *distilled white vinegar* to preserve your solution. Use the same amount of vinegar as you would brandy for proper preservation. Also, you can dilute essence concentrates (the bottle from the set, not the solution of several essences that you just made), five drops in eight ounces of juice or water, and the brandy will be tasteless.

Follow-Up Testing

Often the completion of a situation or process we might be involved in will require a series of flower essences. For example, after doing the basic test, you found that you needed two essences for three days, two times a day. On the day following the completion of this dosage, retest for essences to find out if a new dosage is needed. You may discover that you now need one essence for two days, two times a day. Once this is completed, test again. Keep doing this testing each time you have completed a dosage cycle until you test that no other essences are needed. This means that you are clear, and that either the process has completed or your balance is holding well as you move through the remainder of the cycle.

The issue of follow-up testing is vital to the successful use of flower essences. Frequently I find that people are willing to do the first test, especially when they are not feeling well. They take the needed essences as prescribed and rave about how much better they feel. Then they don't do the follow-up testing, and often the result is that they slip right back into feeling lousy. Just as there are stages in the recuperation period, there are corresponding stages in the flower essences needed. And sometimes the lousy feelings may be completely gone and we think we have come to the end, but we still test the need for essences. This just means we're still in the recuperation period, and despite all evidence to the contrary, it hasn't ended yet. In short, it's important to follow through with the testing all the way to the end.

One other thing to caution you about: Let's say you just got rid of a bad cold. You did all the follow-up testing and you finally tested clear—no other essences needed. Everything is going well for about five days and then you start to feel the cold coming back. As soon as you get those first signs, go right back to testing the essences. This does not mean you made an error in the previous series of tests. Most likely it means that something unexpected has happened in your life and, while in that vulnerable period right after being sick, it just broadsided you, breaking or overloading your electrical circuitry again. If you move quickly with the essences, you'll reestablish the balance and prevent your getting sick again. However, if you do get sick again, keep testing the essences as you move through it until you test clear.

Keeping Records

This is for the people who want to find out more about themselves. Keep a record of the date, the illness or situation, the symptoms you feel, and the essences needed plus dosage. This is especially helpful during that first year or so of using the essences. Eventually you'll be able to look over the record and see what reactions and types of situations result in what symptoms—what situation tends to be the underlying cause of our headaches, or our lower backache, or our sinus trouble. It's another way of discovering personal patterns. If we know that whenever we got a sinus headache we tended to need Zinnia Essence (reconnects one to the child within; restores playfulness, laughter, joy, and a sense of healthy priorities), we can reexamine our life in light of the priorities we choose and our somber attitude, and make some changes that would strike a better balance for us. This would then break the personal patterning that results in sinus headaches. So besides using flower essences to pull us out of each sinus headache, we can use them to begin eliminating the sinus headache cycle altogether.

Surrogate Testing

There may be times when you feel that someone else could be helped by flower essences but does not have them available or is unable to test himself—a child, someone ill, a troubled friend. You can help that person by testing for the essences using a kinesiology surrogate technique, which is also quite simple.

1. *Test yourself first* and take any needed flower essences to make sure you are clear before testing anyone else.

2. Physically make contact with the person you are going to test. Have him place a hand on your knee or touch your foot with his foot. Focus on the person for a

few seconds. This touching and focusing connects his electrical system to yours. Test your connection using the kinesiology technique, asking (aloud or to yourself) if you are fully connected to this person's electrical system. If negative, spend a few more seconds focusing on the individual. If either of you is being distracted, move to a quieter room or quiet the environment you are in. Encourage the other person to keep his mind focused on the hand (or foot) that is touching you. A wandering mind will cause fuzzy test results.

3. If the test for your connection to the other person was positive, you are ready to test for the flower essences. Place the bottles (or box of bottles) in your lap and ask:

Does he/she need any of these flower essences? (Test.)

If positive, place each bottle one at a time in *your* lap and ask if that flower essence is needed. A positive test response indicates that this particular flower essence rebalances the other person's system and makes it strong. (Remember, you have already cleared yourself of any need for the essences prior to starting the surrogate testing.) Double-check your results by placing the needed bottles in the free hand or lap of the person, and ask again if these are the flower essences needed.

If negative, make sure your connection with this person is still positive. Ask:

Am I fully connected to his/her electrical system?

If not, go back to step 2, refocus on the person, and do the testing over again.

If you are connected, retest the other essences to find what was missed. Ask again:

Are these all the essences needed? (Test.)

If the response is positive or only one bottle is needed, go on to step 4.

If negative, you're still missing an essence. Keep retesting the other essences until you get a positive response to the question.

For a combination, place the combination of bottles in the person's free hand or lap, and ask:

Is this the combination he/she needs? (Test.)

If negative, adjust the combination by removing any unnecessary essences. Test each bottle separately by having the person hold it and asking:

Is this bottle needed in the combination? (Test.)

Whatever tests negative gets removed. Check the new combination by asking:

Is this combination now correct? (Test.)

Continue working with the combination until it tests positive.

4. When the needed flower essence(s) has been determined, test for how many days/weeks and how many times a day, using the same yes/no testing procedure you used on yourself. *It is important that you remain physically connected with the other person throughout the entire testing process.*

5. Administer the flower essences needed either

directly on the tongue or in a glass of water. Or, fix a dosage bottle. Test to make sure the person is now clear. Rarely will you get a negative on this. As when testing yourself, a negative result means the person is ready for the Peeling Process. If you and the person would like to continue, immediately refer to the Peeling Process steps in Chapter 8 of *Flower Essences*. However, if you or the other person don't wish to go on to the Peeling Process right away, test for dosage with the essences that just tested positive, and give them to the person.

6. An important component of the effectiveness of all flower essences is understanding. Therefore make sure that whenever possible the person you are working with knows what flower essences are needed and how they are each defined.

Telegraph Testing

The telegraph testing procedure is an important tool to develop and have at hand. It allows you to use flower essences with pinpoint accuracy, and by using telegraph testing along with the basic testing procedure, you can move through symptoms or specific focuses with lightning speed.

When telegraph testing, you are not testing one specific focus or symptom *in relationship to the whole*. That is what you accomplished when you did the basic testing. Instead, you are testing the one thing *on its own in relationship to nothing else*. Consequently, when we find the need for the same essence we just took as a result of the basic test, it is because the symptom or focus itself requires a direct infusion of that essence. Taking it in regard to the overall picture didn't do the trick. (For more information on telegraph testing and the different ways it can be used, see Chapter 8 in the book *Flower Essences*.)

1. Do the basic essence test and take the needed essences. Make sure you are clear from the basic test before going on.

If you test for no essences, do the telegraph testing anyway. Not needing essences for the basic test but needing them for the more specific telegraph test is not unusual and demonstrates why telegraph testing is so effective.

2. Focus on the thing/symptom you wish to test. Make sure your focus is strong, clear, and that you keep that focus throughout the test.

3. While maintaining the focus, test the essences as you would for a basic test. In short, you are doing a regular basic test while maintaining your focus on a specific issue or symptom.

4. Do this testing for each symptom or issue you wish to test. Be sure to take any needed essences, and check for dosage for each telegraph test before moving on to the next test.

5. If you are testing several symptoms or issues, you

may end up with a solution dosage for each. While taking each solution, according to its dosage, you will need to focus again on the specific symptom or issue the solution is addressing.

6. You can do surrogate telegraph testing. *First, you must clear yourself by doing a basic test and taking any needed essences.* Then, set up to do a surrogate basic test. Do the basic test for the person first, and let them take the needed essences. This clears that person. (*It is vital that a person be cleared with the basic test before doing any telegraph testing.*) Follow the surrogate testing steps while you or the person you are working with maintains a focus on the specific issue or symptom.

Appendix D

About Perelandra
and My Research
with Nature

Perelandra is both home for Clarence and me and a nature research center. It now consists of forty-five acres of open fields and woods in the foothills of the Blue Ridge Mountains in Virginia. The nature research and development has been going on since 1976, when I dedicated myself to learning about nature in new ways from nature itself. I began working with nature intelligences in a coordinated, co-creative, and educational effort that has resulted in understanding and demonstrating a new approach to agriculture and ecological balance. Besides publishing materials about the research, we hold an annual workshop series and open house at Perelandra. *Except for these scheduled days, Perelandra is closed to the public in order to have the time and space needed for the continuing research work.* Write us at Perelandra for information about the workshops and open houses.

The primary focus of my work has been the one-hundred-foot-diameter circular garden where I get from nature the information and direction I need to create an all-inclusive garden environment based on the principles of balance. For example, we do not attempt to repel insects. Instead, we focus on creating a balanced environment that calls to it and fully supports a complete and appropriate population of insects. In turn, the insects relate to the garden's plant life in a light and nondestructive manner.

From this work has developed a new method of gardening that I call "co-creative gardening." Briefly, this is a method of gardening in partnership with the nature intelligences that emphasizes balance and teamwork. The balance is a result of concentrating on the laws of nature and form. The teamwork is established between the individual and the intelligent levels inherent in nature. Both of these point out the differences between co-creative agriculture, and traditional organic gardening and agricultural methods. (Information about this work is described in three books: *Behaving As If the God In All Life Mattered*; *Perelandra Garden Workbook: A Complete Guide to Gardening with Nature Intelligences*; and *Perelandra Garden Workbook II: Co-Creative Energy Processes for Gardening, Agriculture and Life.*)

The foundation of the work going on at Perelandra, as I have indicated, comes from nature intelligences, a collective term I use for devas and nature spirits. My work with flower essences and a number of physical health and balancing processes has also been directed from these levels. The following is brief description of these two levels based on how I experience them.

"Deva" is a Sanskrit word used to describe the intelligent level of consciousness within nature that functions in an architectural mode within all that is form and also serves as the organizer of all that is a part of each form. This means that if I should want to understand or change something in the botanical makeup of a plant species, I would consult with the deva of that species for clarification regarding my specific questions and for advice as to whether my change is viable and ecologically sound. The deva of each type of plant holds the architectural blueprints of that plant and has the power to change the blueprints at any time.

"Nature spirit" refers to the intelligent level of consciousness within nature that works in partnership with the devic level and is responsible for the fusing and maintaining of energy to appropriate form. Nature spirits tend to the shifting of an energy reality that has been formulated on the devic level and assist the translation of that reality into form. They also function in a custodial capacity with all that is form on the planet.

To help you understand the work at Perelandra and why nature plays an important and direct role in our health and well-being in general, and MAP and the Calibration Process specifically, I include in Appendix E definitions that were given to me by nature in a coning session. I feel that once you read them you'll sense nature's important role in human health more clearly.

Appendix E

Co-Creative Definitions by Nature and Friends

Let us give you the basic understanding of these terms. We feel that these definitions, kept short and simple, will be more helpful than lengthy, detailed ones. Consider these definitions to be starting points.

✳ **FORM:** *We consider reality to be in the form state when there is order, organization, and life vitality combined with a state of consciousness. For the purpose of understanding form in a constructive and workable manner, let us say that we consider consciousness to be soul-initiated and, therefore, quite capable of function beyond what we would term "form." There are dimensions of reality in which the interaction of life reality is maintained beyond form only. There is no surrounding organization, order, or life vitality as we know it. There is only reality beyond form.*

We do not consider form to be only that which is perceptible to the five senses. In fact, we see form from this perspective to be most limited, both in its life reality and in its ability to function. We see form from the perspective of the five senses to be useful only for the most basic and fundamental level of

301

identification. From this perspective, there is very little relationship to the full understanding and knowledge of how a unit or form system functions.

*All energy contains order, organization, and life vitality; therefore, **all energy is form**. If one were to use the term "form" to identify that which can be perceived by the basic senses and the word "energy" to refer to that aspect of an animal, human, plant, or object's reality that cannot be readily perceived by the basic senses, then one would be accurate in the use of these two words. However, if one were to use the word "form" to refer to that which can be perceived by the basic five senses and assume form to be a complete unit of reality unto itself, and use the word "energy" to refer to a level beyond form, one would then be using these two words inaccurately.*

On the planet Earth, the personality, character, emotional makeup, intellectual capacity, strong points, and gifts of a human are all form. They are that which gives order, organization, and life vitality to consciousness.

Order and organization are the physical structures that create a framework for form. In short, they define the walls. But we have included the dynamic of life vitality when we refer to form because one of the elements of form is action, and it is the life vitality that initiates and creates action.

❋ **NATURE:** *In the larger universe and beyond, on its many levels and dimensions, there are a number of groups of consciousnesses that, although equal in importance, are quite different in expression and function. Do not misunderstand us by thinking that we are saying that all reality is human soul-*

302

oriented but that there are some aspects of this reality that function and express differently. We are not saying this. We are saying that there are different groups of consciousnesses that are equal in importance but express and function very differently. Together, they make up the full expression of the larger, total life picture. No one piece, no one expression, can be missing or the larger life picture on all its levels and dimensions will cease to exist. One such consciousness has been universally termed "nature." Because of what we are saying about the larger picture not existing without all of its parts, you may assume that nature as both a reality and a consciousness exists on all dimensions and all levels. It cannot be excluded.

Each group of consciousnesses has what can be termed an area of expertise. As we said, all groups are equal in importance but express and function differently from one another. These different expressions and functions are vital to the overall balance of reality. A truly symbiotic relationship exists among the groups and is based on balance—universal balance. You are absolutely correct to characterize the human soul-oriented dynamic as evolution in scope and function. And you are correct in identifying the nature dynamic as being involution in scope and function. Nature is a massive, intelligent consciousness group that expresses and functions within the many areas of involution, that is, moving soul-oriented consciousness into any dimension or level of form.

Nature is the conscious reality that supplies order, organization, and life vitality for this shift. Nature is the consciousness that is, for your working understanding, intimately linked with form. Nature is the consciousness that comprises all form on all levels and dimensions. It is form's order, organization, and life vitality. Nature is first and foremost a consciousness of equal importance with all other consciousnesses in the largest scheme of reality. It expresses and functions uniquely in that it comprises all form on all levels and dimensions and is responsible for and creates all of form's order, organization, and life vitality.

✳ **DEVAS AND NATURE SPIRITS:** *"Devas" and "nature spirits" are names used to identify two different expressions and functions within the nature consciousness. They are the two groups within the larger nature consciousness that interface with the human soul while in form. There are other groups, and they are differentiated from one another primarily by specific expression and function.*

To expand from our definition of form, it is the devic expression that fuses with consciousness to create order, organization, and life vitality. The devic expression as the architect designs the complex order, organization, and life vitality that will be needed by the soul consciousness while functioning within the scope or band of form. If the consciousness chooses to shift from one point of form to another point, thereby changing form function, it is the devic expression of nature that alters the organization, order, and life vitality accordingly. The devic expression designs and is the creation of the order, organization, and life vitality of form.

The nature spirit expression infuses the devic order, organization, and life vitality and adds to this the dynamic of function and working balance. To order, organization, and life vitality it brings movement and the bond that maintains the alignment of the devic form unit to the universal principles of balance while the consciousness is in form.

*To say that nature is the expert in areas of form and form principles barely scratches the surface of the true nature (pardon the pun) of nature's role in form. It is the expert of form, and it is form itself. A soul-oriented consciousness cannot exist on any level or dimension of form in any way without an **equal**, intimate, symbiotic relationship with the nature consciousness.*

✳ **CONSCIOUSNESS:** *The concept of consciousness has been vastly misunderstood. To put it simply, consciousness is the working state of the soul. In human expression, as one sees it demonstrated on the planet Earth, the personality, character, emotional makeup, intellectual capacity, strong points, and gifts of a human are all form. They are that which gives order, organization, and life vitality to consciousness.*

We say "working state of the soul" because there are levels of soul existence that are different than the working state and can best be described as a simple and complete state of being. The closest that souls on Earth come to this notion is the state of unconsciousness. But this is to give you a glimpse of what we mean by "state of being." We urge you not to assume that what you know as unconsciousness is equal to the soul state of being.

Humans tend to think of the soul as being something that exists far away from them because they are in form. This is an illusion. The core of any life is the soul. It cannot exist apart from itself. Like the heart in the human body, it is an essential part of the life unit. A human in form is, by definition, a soul fused with nature. Personality and character are a part of the nature/form package that allows the soul to function and to express itself in form. They are not the soul; they are the order and organization of that soul.

Consciousness physically fuses into the body system first through the electrical system and then through the central nervous system and the brain. This is another aspect of nature supplying order, organization, and life vitality. Consciousness itself cannot be measured or monitored as a reality. But what can be measured and monitored is the order, organization, and life vitality of consciousness. Consciousness is the working state of the soul and is not form. It is nature, not consciousness, that supplies form.

We wish to add a thought here so that there will be no confusion about the relationship between nature and the soul. The devic level of nature does not, with its own power, superimpose its interpretation of form onto a soul. We have said that nature and soul are intimately and symbiotically related. This implies a give and take. No one consciousness group operates in isolation of the whole or of all other parts of the whole. When a soul chooses to move within the vast band of form, it communicates its intent and purpose to nature. It is from this that nature, on the devic level, derives the specifics that will be needed for the soul to function in form. It is a perfect marriage of purpose with the order, organization, and life vitality that is needed for the fulfillment of that purpose. Nature, therefore, does not define purpose and impose it on a *soul. It orders, organizes, and gives life vitality to purpose for expression of form.*

✳ **SOUL:** *We perceive that most likely the question of soul will arise with anyone reading these definitions. This will be most difficult to define since the soul is, at its point of central essence, beyond form. Consequently, it is beyond words. However, it is not beyond any specific life form. As we have said, an individual is not separate or distant from his or her soul. Souls, as individuated life forces, were created in form at the moment you call the "Big Bang." Beyond form, souls are also beyond the notion of creation. So we refer to the moment of the Big Bang regarding the soul, since this gives you a description of soul that will be most meaningful to you.*

The Big Bang was the nature-designed order, organization, and life force used to differentiate soul into sparks of individuated light energy. The power of the Big Bang was created by intent. And that intent originated from the massive collective soul reality beyond form.

It is reasonable to look at the Big Bang as the soul's gateway to the immense band of form. To perceive the soul and how it functions exclusively from the perspective of human form on Earth is akin to seeing that planet from the perspective of one grain of sand. The soul's options of function and expression in form are endless. What we see occurring more frequently now on Earth is the shift from the individual soul unknowingly functioning in an array of options, all chosen only because they are compatible to the immediate purpose of the soul, to the individual beginning to function with discrimination and intent in more expanded ways. Using the words in their more limited, parochial definitions, we can say that we see the beginning of a shift from soul function in which an individuated personality remains unaware of many of its options to soul function in which the personality begins to take on conscious awareness of all its options.

✳ **ENERGY:** *For those experiencing life on Earth, energy is form that is perceived by an individual beyond the scope of the basic five senses. All energy contains order, organization, and life vitality; therefore, **all energy is form**. The makeup and design of the specific order, organization, and life vitality within that which can be perceived by the basic five senses is identical to and therefore harmonious with its broader reality, which cannot be perceived by the basic five senses. If one is to use the term "form" to identify that which can be perceived by the basic senses and the word "energy" to refer to that aspect of an animal, human, plant, or object's reality that cannot be readily perceived by the basic senses, then one would be accurate in the use of these two words. However, if one is to use the word "form" to refer to that which can be perceived by the basic five senses and assume form to be a complete unit of reality unto itself, and use the word "energy" to refer to a level beyond form, one would then be using these two words inaccurately. From our perspective, form and energy create one unit of reality and are differentiated from one another solely by the individual's ability to perceive them with his or her sensory system. In short, the differentiation between that which is form and that which is energy within any given object, plant, animal, or human lies with the observer.*

✳ **BASIC SENSORY SYSTEM PERCEPTION:** *We define basic sensory system perception as being that which the vast majority of individuals on Earth experience. The acts of seeing, hearing, touching, tasting, and smelling fall within what we acknowledge as a basic, fundamental range of sensory development that is predominant on the Earth level. What is referred to as an "expansion experience" is, in fact, an act or experience that is perceived by an individual because of an expansion of the range in which his sensory system operates. Expansion experiences are not perceived outside or beyond an individual's electrical system, central nervous system, and sensory system. These three systems are interrelated, and an accurate perception of an expansion experience requires that the three systems operate in concert. Therefore, it is quite possible for something to occur in an individual's life that registers in the person's electrical system and central nervous system but then short-circuits, is altered, or is blocked simply because the person's present sensory system does not have the ability to process, due to its present range of operation, what has registered in the other two systems. People say that "these kinds of strange things never happen to me." This is inaccurate. "Strange" things, experiences, and moments beyond the present state of their sensory systems are continuously happening around them and to them. They are simply not at the point where their sensory systems are capable of clear, useful processing. They waste time by directing their will and focus to "make things happen." That is useless since things are happening all the time around them. Instead they should relax and continue through an organic developmental process* *that is already in effect and that will gradually allow them to accurately perceive what is happening around them. In some cases where events or experiences are vaguely perceived or processed in outrageous, useless ways, their sensory system is expanding but still not operating within the range where events can be usefully processed.*

✳ **REALITY:** *From our perspective, reality refers to all levels and dimensions of life experience within form and beyond form. Reality does not depend on an individual's perception of it in order to exist. We call an individual's perception of reality his "perceived reality." Any life system that was created in form (which occurred at the moment of the Big Bang) has inherent in it all dimensions and levels that exist both within form and beyond. How we relate to an individual or object depends on our present ability to enfold and envelop an individual's many levels. The scope within which one exists, the reality of one's existence, is truly beyond form, beyond description. If one understands that the evolutionary force that moves all life systems forward is endless—beyond time—then one must also consider that it is the continuous discovery of these vast levels inherent in all life systems that creates that evolutionary momentum. Since that dynamic is beyond time as expressed on any form level or dimension, it is endless.*

✳ **PERCEIVED REALITY:** *This is the combination of elements that make up an individual's full system of reality and are perceived, embraced, and enfolded by him or by another individual at any given time. From this, an individual "knows" himself or another individual only from the perspec-*

tive of the specific combination of elements he or she is able to perceive, embrace, and enfold. Any one element can be considered a window to the larger whole. When in form, these elements take on the dynamics of order, organization, and life vitality and are demonstrated through these specific form frameworks. The extent to which perceived reality corresponds to the larger, all-encompassing reality depends on the ability of an individual to accurately demonstrate these elements within form frameworks and the ability of that or another individual to accurately perceive what is being demonstrated.

✳ **BALANCE:** *Balance is relative and measured, shall we say, by an individual's ability to faithfully demonstrate the various elements that make up his larger reality through the specific frameworks of form in which one has chosen to develop. When what one is demonstrating is faithful in intent and clarity with these elements and the larger reality, one experiences balance. And those interacting with this individual will experience his balance. One experiences imbalance when there is distortion between what one demonstrates through the form framework and the intent and clarity of the elements that make up the larger reality as well as the larger reality itself.*

If you seriously consider what we are saying here, you will see that balance as a phenomenon is not an elusive state that only an exalted few can achieve. Balance is, in fact, inherent in all reality, in all life systems. Balance is defined by the many elements within any individual's reality. And it is the dominant state of being within any reality and any form system. It is also the state of being that links individual life systems to one another and to the larger whole. When one says

311

that he is a child of the universe, what one is acknowledging is the relationship and link of his higher state of balance to the universe's state of balance. Whether he feels linked to or distant from this relationship depends on the closeness or distance he creates within himself with respect to his larger personal state of balance—that dynamic that is part of his overall reality.

✳ **LIFE VITALITY:** *We have used this term frequently in these definitions and feel it would be useful to clarify what we mean. To understand life vitality, it is best to see it in relationship to order and organization. Order and organization are the physical structures that create the framework for form. In short, they define the walls. But we have included the dynamic of life vitality when we refer to form because one element of form is action, and it is life vitality that initiates and creates action. Nothing in form is stagnant. It is life vitality that gives to form its action. If the framework that is created from order and organization is incomplete, ineffective, deteriorating or being dismantled in an untimely manner, the dynamic of life vitality decreases within the overall form reality. This causes life movement to decrease accordingly, and is a movement toward a state of stagnation. It is the dynamic of vitality that gives life—movement—to any individual or object. Organization and order alone cannot do that. However, vitality without organization and order has no sense of purpose to its motion. It cannot function without organization and order. The three must be present and in balance with one another for there to be quality form expression. Nature, on the devic level, creates organization, order, and life vitality in perfect balance.*

Nature, on the nature spirit level, maintains that balanced relationship as individual life units move through their evolutionary paces.

We would like to illustrate what we are saying by focusing your attention on the soil-balancing process that improves and enhances the level of soil vitality. This process does not work directly with the soil's vitality level. Instead, it works with those elements of the soil that constitute its order and organization. The process shores up the physical structure of its order and organization. As a direct result, the soil begins to shift its form back to the original balance among organization, order, and life vitality. As a consequence of this shift, the soil vitality level (the soil's life vitality) increases to its new state of balance. Those changes involve a comparable shift in the interaction and movement among all the different elements that make up soil. This is why when someone observes change in a field that has had its soil balanced through the soil-balancing process, he sees greater efficiency between how the soil and plants interact. The action and movement in the soil have raised the soil's order and organizational structures back to the state (or nearer to the state) of the original devic balance of order, organization, and life vitality.

❋ GROUNDING: *Quite simply, the word "grounded" is used to acknowledge full body/soul fusion or full matter/soul fusion. The word "grounding" refers to what must be accomplished or activated in order to both ensure and stabilize body or matter/soul fusion. To be grounded refers to the state of being a fused body (matter)/soul unit. To achieve this unit fusion and to function fully as a fused unit is the primary goal one accepts when choosing to experience life within form. Functioning as a grounded body (matter)/soul unit is a goal on all levels and dimensions of form, whether the form can or cannot be perceived by the five senses.*

Nature plays two key roles in grounding. First, it is through and with nature that the grounding occurs. Nature, which organizes, orders, and adds life vitality to create form, is what creates and maintains grounding. Second, the levels of nature know what is required to fuse the soul dynamic within form. Nature provides the best examples of body (matter)/soul fusion. Humans have recognized the form or matter existence of nature on the planet, but have only recently begun to understand that within all form there are fully functioning soul dynamics. On the other hand, humans acknowledge or concentrate on their personal soul dynamics but have little understanding as to how they, in order to be functional within form, must allow the soul to fuse with and operate through their form body. Humans do not see the examples or learn the lessons of the master teachers of body (matter)/soul fusion that surround them in all the kingdoms of nature. Humans also deny the fusion within themselves. The relative extent of this denial interferes proportionately with the quality and stabilization of the fusion.

✴ **INTENT:** *Intent refers to the conscious dynamic within all life that links life vitality with soul purpose and direction. When an individual uses free will to manipulate what he or she willfully desires instead of what is within the scope of higher soul purpose, then intent is combined with the manipulative power of free will and this combination is linked*

314

with life vitality. If you will recall, it is life vitality that adds action to order and organization. It both initiates and creates action. To maintain harmonious movement with soul purpose and direction, life vitality must be linked with the soul dynamic. This linkage occurs on two levels. One is unconscious, allowing for a natural patterning and rhythm of action through form that is consistent with soul purpose. As the body/soul fusion moves through its own evolutionary process as a functioning unit, it takes on a greater level of consciousness and an expanded level of awareness and knowing. As a result, the unconscious link between soul dynamic and life vitality takes on a new level of operation, thus shifting it into a state of consciousness. The shift is a gradual, step-by-step evolutionary process in itself. Intent is conscious awareness of soul purpose, what is required within the scope of form to achieve soul purpose, and how the two function as a unit. Consequently, when one wishes to express soul purpose, one need only consciously fuse this purpose with appropriate form and action. This act is what is referred to when one speaks of intent.

Intent as a dynamic is an evolutionary process in itself and, as we have said, does not suddenly envelop one's entire life fully and completely. Intent is only gradually incorporated into one's everyday life. Therefore, one does not suddenly and immediately function within the full scope of the intent dynamic in those areas of life where intent is present. Intent as a dynamic is as broad a learning arena as life itself. And in the beginning, intent can often be confused with or intermingled with free will. However, as it is developed, it becomes the cutting edge of the body/soul unit and how it operates. Intent is the key to unlimited life within the scope of form.

✳ **INTUITION:** *Intuition, as it is popularly defined, relates to a sixth sense of operation. This is false. This is not a sixth sense. When individuals experience a phenomenon that they consider to be beyond their five senses, they tend to attribute this experience to another category, the sixth sense, and call it intuition. The fact is that these expanded experiences are processed through their five senses in an expanded manner.*

Intuition, in fact, is related to and linked with intent. It is the bridge between an individual's conscious body/soul fusion—that state which he knows and understands about the body/soul fusion and how it functions—and the individual's unconscious body/soul fusion. The intuition bridges the unconscious and the conscious. This enables what is known on the level of the unconscious body/soul fusion to be incorporated with and become a part of the conscious body/soul fusion. Intuition is the communication bridge between the two that makes it possible for the conscious body/soul unit to benefit from those aspects of the unconscious body/soul unit. This benefit results when the conscious unit opens to and moves through the lessons surrounding intent. Where intent is functioning fully, these two levels, the unconscious and the conscious, are no longer separate but have become one—the expanded conscious level. Consequently, there is then no need for the bridge known as intuition.

However, lest you think otherwise, intent is not considered greater than intuition; rather, they are two excellent tools utilized equally by the highest developed souls functioning within

316

form. We say this to caution those who read this not to think intent is "greater" than intuition and to be aimed for at the exclusion of intuition. Evolution as seen from the highest perspective is endless. Therefore, discovery of all there is to know about both intuition and intent is endless. For all practical purposes, an individual can safely consider that there will never be a time in which the development of intent will be such that the need for and development of intuition will be unnecessary. As we have said, the highest souls who function to the fullest within the scope of form do so with an equal development and expansion of both intent and intuition.

A MESSAGE TO MAP USERS: This past year we have become aware of several people who are running around telling people that there is a "new MAP," and they just happen to be the one chosen to inform everyone about the MAP changes. They've even said that the MAP teams haven't yet told me about the changes. Then they proceed to scare the bejeesus out of people by telling them things like they are being attacked and taken over by aliens and the MAP teams want them to keep their coning open twenty-four hours a day for the rest of their lives. Here are some facts about MAP that I hope will put you at ease.

1. The head of the MAP program is Lorpuris, the head of the White Brotherhood Medical Unit. I generally speak with him daily. He's not going to change the MAP program without telling me about it. It's not as if we don't talk to one another and he hasn't gotten around to telling me this little bit of news.

2. MAP has a built-in protection. It was decided prior to the program "going public" that any modifications or changes would come through Perelandra. This is not because we at Perelandra claim a monopoly on MAP. It is to avoid confusion among MAP users. Without this coordination anyone could announce changes to the program, and everyone would have to figure out whose changes were legitimate and whose were not, creating a fair amount of chaos in the program. This has been eliminated by coordinating a "centralized information hub" at Perelandra.

3. MAP was designed to accommodate the wide range of approaches that are needed for the many different people who participate in the program. In part, this was done so that the teams would not have to modify the program for a long time. MAP has not become obsolete and the teams do not anticipate needing to change it for many years to come.

4. Because MAP is set up to meet individual needs, it is not unusual for one team's approach and work to be quite different from how the other teams work. It is important that we not confuse what is unique about our personal MAP work and think it is what everyone else needs to do or that it is a sign of wholesale changes in the program.

If you know someone who has been "taken in" by would-be MAP changes, suggest to them to go back to using the program as it is outlined in the book. They need to talk to their team about the frustrations they are having with MAP that made them open to suggestions to changing the program in the first place. When someone deliberately attempts to shift the session setup outside the structure of the program, their team will not continue to work with them. Instead, whenever a MAP coning is opened the team will attempt to bring the person back to understanding what MAP is about and stabilize the person until he is ready to participate in the program as it has been set up. No matter how hard a person tries, he cannot manipulate a MAP team to operate in ways the team does not wish to operate.

If you have gotten caught up with someone else's ideas about how MAP should be used and you are still confused after reading this, please write or call us at Perelandra so that we can help you get back on track.

MAP Order Form

A complete listing of all Perelandra products is included in our free catalog, which is sent upon request. Prices in this order form are subject to change.

___ *Behaving as if the God in All Life Mattered* (1997 edition) $12.95 *
___ *Dancing in the Shadows of the Moon* (hardcover) $23
___ *Perelandra Garden Workbook* (second edition) $19.95
___ *Perelandra Garden Workbook II* $16.95
___ *Flower Essences* $10.95
      (When purchased with any set of Perelandra Essences: $8)
___ *MAP* (second edition) $14.95 *
___ *Perelandra Microbial Balancing Program Manual* $16
___ *Co-Creative Science* $11

___ Perelandra Paper # 4: Body/Soul Fusion Process $2

* These books are also available in Spanish, see the Perelandra catalog for details.

Perelandra Essences

___ **Basic Set:** Rose I & Garden Essences (1/2-oz. bottles) $102
___ **Basic Dram Set:** Rose I & Garden Essences (1/8-oz. bottles) $74

___ **Expanded Set:** Rose I, Garden & Rose II (1/2-oz. bottles) $136
___ **Expanded Dram Set:** Rose I, Garden & Rose II (1/8-oz. bottles) $95

___ **All Essences 1:** Rose I, Garden & Rose II (dram bottles), Nature
      Program & Soul Ray Essences (1/2-oz. bottles) $173
___ **All Essences 2:** Rose I, Garden, Rose II, Nature Program &
      Soul Ray Essences (1/2-oz. bottles only) $214

___ Perelandra Rose I Essences Set (1/2-oz. bottles only) $40
___ Perelandra Garden Essences Set (1/2-oz. bottles only) $78
___ Perelandra Rose Essences II Set (1/2-oz bottles only) $40
___ Perelandra Nature Program Essences Set (1/2-oz. bottles only) $47
      (When purchased with an Expanded Set of essences: $42)
___ Perelandra Soul Ray Essences Set (1/2-oz. bottles only) $42
      (When purchased with an Expanded Set of essences: $37)

___ Individual Rose I, Garden & Rose II Essences
      (1/2-oz. bottles only) $6.50 ea.   (List below.)

U.S. Postage & Handling (See catalog for international rates.)

thru $8 . . . . $2.20

$8.01 to 14.00 . . . . $4.00

$14.01 to 25.00 . . . . . . $5.00

$25.01 to 50.00 . . . . . . $6.00

$50.01 to 75.00 . . . . . . $7.30

$75.01 to 100.00. . . . . . $8.30

$100.01 to 200.00. . . . . $9.40

$200.01 to $300.00. . . . $11.50

$300.01 & over . . . . . . 5% of order

AK, HI, VI & PR: If your subtotal is over $50, please send 1-½ times this domestic chart. (Package will be shipped by first class mail.)

Prices and shipping charges are subject to change without notice.

Subtotal _____		
Postage & Handling _____		
VA residents only: + 4.5% sales tax _____		
Total _____		

☐ *Please preserve my essences in distilled white vinegar instead of brandy.*

☐ *Send additional catalog(s). Quantity:* _____

Method of Payment:

☐ Check/Money Order ☐ Visa ☐ MasterCard ☐ Discover

Please print more clearly than you ever have in your entire life.

Name _____

UPS Address _____

_____

City _____

State & Zip _____

Daytime Phone _____

Card Number _____

Expiration Date _____ / _____ / _____

Signature _____

Credit card orders must be accompanied by signature.

Perelandra, Ltd. ❧ P.O. Box 3603, Warrenton, VA 20188

U.S./Canada: 1-800-960-8806 ❧ Overseas/Mexico: 1-540-937-2153

Fax: 1-540-937-3360 ❧ http://www.perelandra-ltd.com